ALLE · ZEIT · WACH · 1842

N. Heyder E. G. Hahn B. B. Goldberg (Eds.)

Innovations in Abdominal Ultrasound

With 102 Figures, Some in Color

Springer-Verlag
Berlin Heidelberg New York
London Paris Tokyo
Hong Kong Barcelona
Budapest

Prof. Dr. med. Norbert Heyder
Prof. Dr. med. Eckhart G. Hahn
Medizinische Klinik I mit Poliklinik
der Friedrich-Alexander-Universität Erlangen-Nürnberg
Krankenhausstrasse 12, W-8520 Erlangen, FRG

Prof. Dr. med. Barry B. Goldberg
Thomas Jefferson University Hospital, Division of Ultrasound
132 S., 10th Street, Suite 781 G, Philadelphia, PA 19107, USA

ISBN 3-540-55650-8 Springer-Verlag Berlin Heidelberg New York
ISBN 0-387-55650-8 Springer-Verlag New York Berlin Heidelberg

Library of Congress Cataloging-in-Publication Data
Innovations in abdominal ultrasound / N. Heyder, E.G. Hahn, B.B. Goldberg (eds.). Includes bibliographical references and index. ISBN 3-540-55650-8 (alk. paper) – ISBN 0-387-55650-8 (alk. paper) 1. Abdomen – Ultrasonic imaging. 2. Endoscopic ultrasonography. 3. Abdomen – ultrasonography. I. Heyder, N. (Norbert) II. Hahn, E. G. (Eckhart G.) III. Goldberg, Barry B., 1937- . [DNLM: 1. Ultrasonography – methods. 2. Ultrasonography – trends.
WI 900 I575] RC944.I54 1992 617.5′507543 – dc20

Typesetting: Mitterweger Werksatz GmbH, Plankstadt, FRG

19/3130 – 543210 – Printed on acid-free paper

Preface

Since the beginnings of diagnostic ultrasound in the 1950s, each decade has seen significant advances in this technology. Commercialization of ultrasound occurred during the 1960s with the introduction of many of the clinical uses that are in existence today. The 1970s showed the most dramatic changes with the commercial introduction of gray-scale and real-time ultrasound. In the 1980s many new advances were introduced, including color Doppler, as well as a wide variety of endoluminal approaches, including endorectal, endovaginal and transesophageal. The decade of the 1990s promises even more significant advances with further transducer miniaturization, three-dimensional ultrasound, and the introduction of a variety of ultrasound contrast agents.

With such rapid changes occurring, it becomes important to disseminate knowledge in as rapid a fashion as possible, thus it was quite appropriate that a meeting such as this be held to provide an in-depth review of the many new areas of ultrasound imaging that show promise for the future. Emphasis was on the new uses of ultrasound in gastrointestinal diseases. Many of these advances will, of course, also have applications in many other areas of the body. It is hoped that those in attendance will acquire a much broader understanding of where ultrasound is now and where it is headed in the not too distant future.

Philadelphia, USA
and Erlangen, FRG
August 1992

B. B. Goldberg
N. Heyder
E. G. Hahn

Contents

Saccharide-Based Ultrasound Contrast Media: Basic Characteristics and Results of Clinical Trials . 1
R. Schlief, R. Schürmann, and H. P. Niendorf

Ultrasound Backscatter of Liver with Particulate Contrast Agents 8
T. A. Tuthill, R. B. Baggs, M. R. Violante, and K. J. Parker

Diagnosis of Colon Tumors and Inflammatory Large-Bowel Diseases by Hydro-colonic Sonography 16
B. Limberg

Endoscopic Ultrasound: Recent Advances in Gastroenterology 27
M. Fukuda, K. Hirata, M. Mitani, T. Mochizuki, and H. Tatuguchi

Doppler Flowmetry in Portal Hypertension 49
L. Bolondi, S. Gaiani, and L. Barbara

Color Doppler Endosonography in the Study of Portal Hypertension 61
L. Bolondi, S. Gaiani, G. Zironi, F. Fornari, S. Siringo, and L. Barbara

Cystogastric Catheter Drainage of Pancreatic Collections of Fluid Under Endoscopic/Ultrasonographic Guidance . . . 70
N. Heyder, E. Günter, and E. G. Hahn

Tumor Therapy by Ethanol Injection: Results and Indications 79
T. Livraghi

Intravascular Scanning Devices and Their Clinical Value 81
K. Bom, C. T. Lancée, W. J. Gussenhoven, J. Roelandt, W. Li, and M. G. M. de Kroon

Advances in Ultrasound: Contrast Agents and Endoluminal Ultrasound 87
B. B. Goldberg and J.-B. Liu

Possibilities of Three-Dimensional Sonography in Obstetrics 110
A. Kratochwil

Three-Dimensional Volumetric Scans: Acquisition Technique and Volume Content Viewing 119
A. Hesse

Clinical TNM Cancer Staging with Endosonography 127
T. L. Tio

Subject Index 143

List of Authors

Bolondi, Luigi, M. D., Prof.
Clinica Medica Università di Bologna, Policlinico S. Orsola, Via Massarenti 9, 40138 Bologna, Italy

Bom, Klaas, Ph. D., Prof.
University of Rotterdam, Thorax Centre EE 2302, P. O. Box 1738, 3000 DR Rotterdam, The Netherlands

Fukuda, Morimichi, M. D., Prof.
Sapporo Medical College Hospital, Department of Ultrasound and Medicine Electronics, S.1, W.17 Chuo-ku, Sapporo 060, Japan

Goldberg, Barry B., M. D., Prof.
Thomas Jefferson University Hospital, Division of Diagnostic Ultrasound, 132 S 10th Street, Philadelphia, PA 19107, USA

Hesse, Alexander, Dr. Ing.
View Point GmbH, Talhofstr. 30, 8031 Gilching, FRG

Heyder, Norbert, M. D., Prof.
Medizinische Klinik mit Poliklinik, Universität Erlangen-Nürnberg, Krankenhausstr. 12, 8520 Erlangen, FRG

Kratochwil, Alfred, M. D.
Allgemeines Öffentliches Krankenhaus der Kurstadt Baden, Gynäkologie, Wimmergasse 19, 2500 Baden, Austria

Limberg, Bernd, M. D.
Klinik Wolfenbüttel, Abteilung Innere Medizin, Akademisches Lehrkrankenhaus der Universität Göttingen, Alter Weg 80, 3340 Wolfenbüttel/Braunschweig, FRG

Livraghi, Tito, M. D., Prof.
Department of Radiology, Ospedale Civile, 20059 Vimercate (MI), Italy

Schlief, Reinhard, M. D., Dipl.-Phys., Dr. Ing.
Clinical Research Diagnostics, Schering AG, Postfach 65 03 11,
1000 Berlin 65, FRG

Tio, Thian Lok, M. D.
Georgetown-University, Medical Center,
Department of Gastroenterology, 3800 Reservoir Road,
Washington, DC 20072197, USA

Tuthill, Theresa Anne, Ph. D.
Department of Electrical Engineering,
University of Rochester, Rochester, NY 14627, USA

Saccharide-Based Ultrasound Contrast Media: Basic Characteristics and Results of Clinical Trials

R. Schlief, R. Schürmann, and H.P. Niendorf

Introduction

Signal intensity in the image is due to the acoustic backscatter behaviour of the body region under investigation (echogenicity); it also depends on the existence of acoustic inhomogeneities in the micrometer range. Echo-enhancing agents must, therefore provide a sufficiently large and reproducible number of micrometer-sized acoustic scatterers in the body region of diagnostic interest. Following the pioneering work of Gramiak and Shah in 1968 [1], it was reported by Meltzer and coworkers in 1980 [2] that tiny gaseous bubbles (microbubbles), within specially prepared solutions, create the desired echo-enhancing effect in the blood after injection. All industrial developments known so far from publications are based on gaseous microbubbles [3, 4]. Because of their unique acoustic properties, gaseous bubbles therefore play a similar basic role as contrast agents in ultrasound as that played by iodine in X-ray diagnosis and by gadolinium in magnetic resonance imaging.

Without any further stabilisation, microbubbles have a very short life span after intravenous injection. This causes the well-known problems of reproducibility of the echo-enhancing effect of self-made preparations. A further stress test of intravascular bubble stability is pulmonary transit and the creation of an echo-enhancing effect in the left heart cavities and arterial vessels after intravenous injection. Very few currently known agents can do this.

Characteristics of the Saccharide-Based Agents SH U 454 and SH U 508 A

The concept of the saccharide-based contrast agents SH U 454 and SH U 508 A is the same: specially produced galactose microparticles that must be suspended in either watery galactose solution (SH U 454) or sterile water (SH U 508 A) before use. After injection, the microbubble-containing suspension leads to a dose-dependent, sharp increase in blood echogenicity until the tracer microparticles and microbubbles dissolve in the blood stream.

SH U 454 dissolves after dilution before reaching the left heart and therefore may be used for B-mode and Doppler echocardiography of the right heart ("right heart agent") and the venous system. It may also serve as an echogenic indicator solution for investigations of fallopian tube patency.

SH U 508 A displays increased microbubble stability because of a small change in the galenic formulation compared with SH U 454. After intravenous injection it leads to an increase in blood echogenicity which survives pulmonary transit (transpulmonary agent) and finally subsides in the arterial system. The transiently echogenic blood stream permits visualisation of the haemodynamics in B-mode, for example for delineation of endocardial borders, or may be employed to increase the Doppler signal intensity in the whole vascular system.

After intravascular dissolution of the acoustically active microstructures, the remaining tracer compound galactose is degraded mainly in the liver (independently of insulin). Galactose is known to be non-toxic and to have no known allergenic potential. The small total amount of air (about 100 µl) is excreted by respiration.

It is desirable that acoustic contrast agents in the diagnostic dosage range lead only to minor and insignificant changes in the overall acoustic properties of the tissue. Otherwise, scanning artefacts due to change in sound velocity or attenuation may occur. The bubble-containing microparticle suspensions of SH U 454 and SH U 508 A exhibit sound velocities within the range of physiological, values, and in diagnostic concentrations and common transducer frequencies only a minor increase in attenuation can be observed which does not lead to relevant image disturbances.

A peculiarity of bubble agents is the pressure dependency of bubble concentration and bubble diameter and consequently their backscatter properties. As reported recently by Mottley and coworkers [5], bubble agents show an increasing decay of echogenicity with increasing ambient pressure within the range of blood pressure (static conditions). Whereas with the saccharide agent SH U 454 this decay under high pressure needs up to some minutes, with air-filled spheres of sonicated human albumin the decay time is only some seconds. Using pressure changes with physiological frequencies (about 1 Hz) with the saccharide agents a reversible cyclic change in backscatter was found in vitro. This cyclic response shows a good correlation with the values of the ambient pressure amplitudes [6]. Figure 1 shows a linear correlation between a calculated backscatter factor and the pressure amplitudes using SH U 508 A. Whether this behaviour can be used in future for evaluation of pressure curves from contrast images is currently under investigation.

Cavitation phenomena and oscillation of bubbles in the ultrasonic field have been discussed as sources of potential hazards by inducing cell lysis. Using ultrasound of therapeutic intensity values, Williams and coworkers [7] found no increase in lysis of erythrocytes after introducing the microbubble agent Echovist if the haematocrit value exceeded 5.5 %. Only at non-physiological low haematocrit values of 1 % – 2 % did a measurable increase in cell lysis occur.

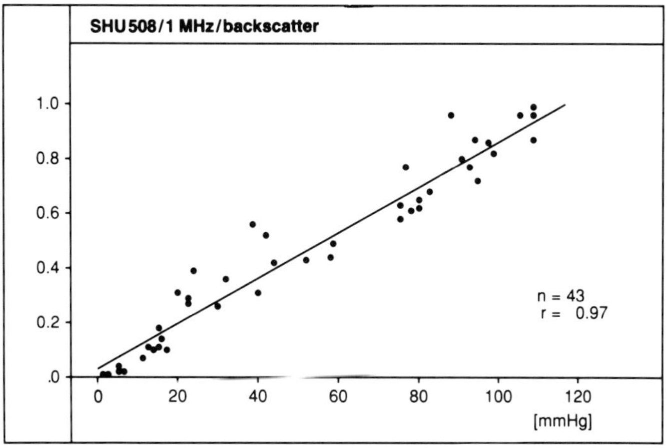

Fig. 1. Correlation between a calculated backscatter factor and physiological pressure amplitudes measured and static conditions

Results of Clinical Trials with SH U 454

The clinical development of SH U 454 is at an advanced stage. In Europe a total of more than 2500 patients have so far been investigated in multicentre trials, with the main indications being echocardiography (B-mode and Doppler; $n > 1850$), venous vessels ($n > 200$) and fallopian tube imaging ($n > 450$).

Representative imaging results of B-mode echocardiography are shown in Fig. 2, colour Doppler in Fig. 3 and transvaginal tubal [8] imaging (hysterosalpingo-contrast sonography) in Fig. 4.

We found good overall tolerance of SH U 454, without any specific risk of severe side effects or clinically relevant changes of circulatory function or blood chemistry after intravenous injections. The only exclusion criteria were galactosaemia or an acute, critical clinical condition of a patient.

Results of Clinical Trials with SH U 508 A

A phase I clinical trial revealed a reproducible and intense opacification of the left ventricle after intravenous injections of SH U 508 and good diagnostic efficacy of the reproducible echo enhancement in the left heart chambers [10]. First clinical trials in patients are continuing and so far include more than 250 patients with various heart diseases in ten European centres. Preliminary results show a good diagnostic efficacy. Figure 5 shows a representative sequence from the on-going phase II studies. Thanks to the previously discussed advantageous acoustic properties of the agent a diagnostic left heart opacification can be obtained after intravenous injection of SH 508 A

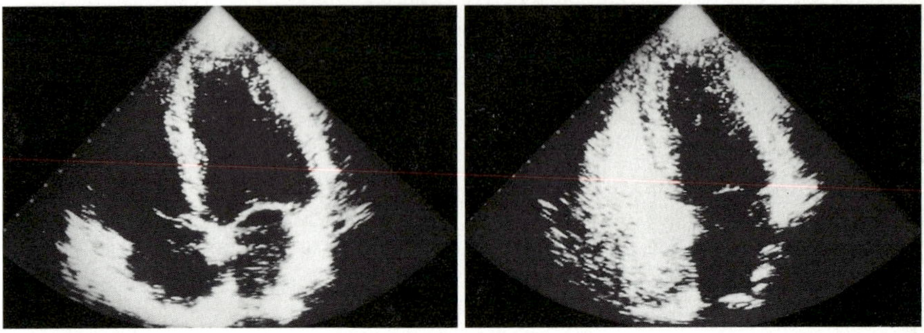

Fig. 2. Echocardiographic apical four-chamber view before *(left)* and after injection of SH U 454 *(right)*. After injection, the echogenically labelled bloodstream can be observed and pathological changes excluded. (From [9])

without relevant imaging artefacts such as shadowing or changes in anatomical shape (Fig. 5a).

Although measureable cyclic changes in echo intensity exist, they do not cause a visible drop-off in systole, as can be seen from the systolic frame shown in Fig. 5d.

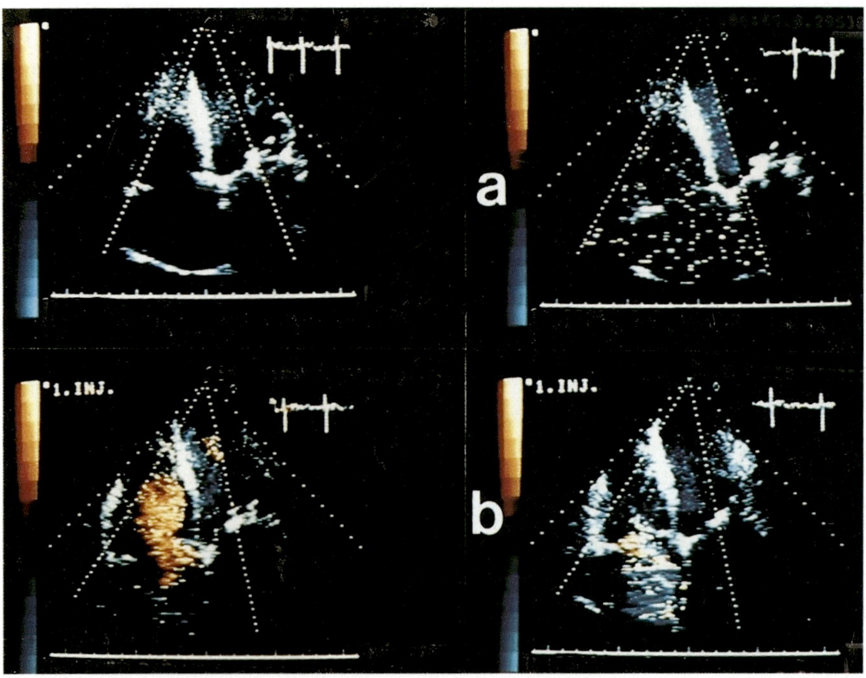

Fig. 3 a, b. Colour flow mapping, four-chamber view before **(a)** and after **(b)** injection of Echovist. (From [9])

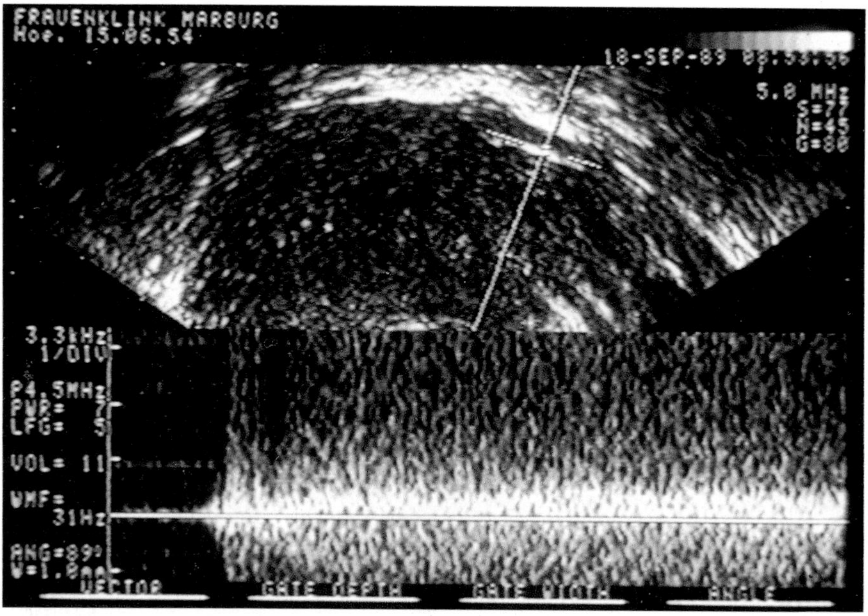

Fig. 4. Duplex hysterosalpingocontrast sonography shows patency of the left fallopian tube. The characteristic noisy Doppler tracing during pertubation helps confirm patency

First patient examinations with contrast-enhanced colour Doppler imaging of the left heart have revealed advantages in cases of suboptimal flow detection in the plain scan, for example, in diagnosing valvular insufficiency. Figure 6 shows a case of mitral regurgitation which was not seen in the plain scan but became visible after intravenous injection of SH U 508 A due to the resultant increase in Doppler signal intensity [11].

In all patients examined to date, the injections of SH U 508 A were well tolerated up to the applied maximum concentration of 400 mg microparticles per 1 ml suspension and the applied maximum volume of 16 ml.

Future Prospects

Initial results of clinical pilot studies have demonstrated advantages of intravenous injections of SH U 508 A in transcranial Doppler examinations, in trans-oesophageal Doppler examinations of coronary blood flow, in stress echocardiography and in vascular Doppler signal enhancement. Future clinical trials will cover hysterosalpingo-contrast sonography and urodynamics.

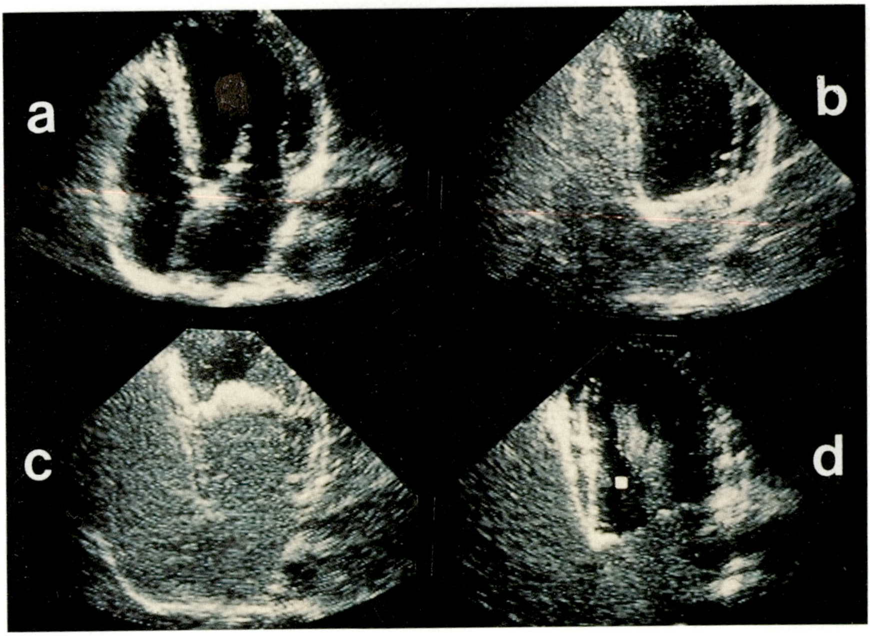

Fig. 5a – d. Echocardiographic apical four-chamber view before **(a)** and after injection of SH U508A **(b, c, d)**. **b** Echogenic contrast flow in the right heart cavities and already arriving in the left atrium after pulmonary transit. **c** First diastolic inflow into the left ventricle. **d** Corresponding end-systolic phase with the echogenically labelled residual blood volume

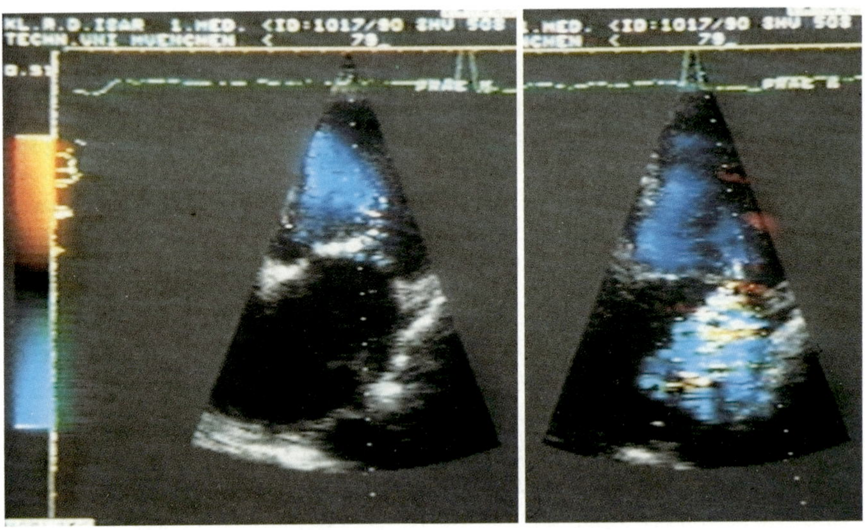

Fig. 6. Echocardiographic color Doppler scan of the leaft heart before *(left)* and after intravenous injection of SH U508A *(right)*. The systolic regurgitation through the mitral valve was not seen in the plain scan *(left)*. After intravenous injection of SH U508A a relevant regurgitant flow becomes visible due to increase in the Doppler signal intensity. (From [11])

Conclusion

The saccharide-based ultrasound contrast agents SH U 454 (Echovist) and SH U 508 A are based chemically on microparticles of the non-toxic tracer compound galactose. Their tolerance as confirmed by broad clinical trials is good. This type of agent represents an advantageous compromise between safety-relevant, sufficient intravascular dissolution rate and diagnostically adequate in vivo stability. Furthermore, they have only a low potential for producing acoustic artefacts in the diagnostic dosage range and exhibit only a low amplitude pressure sensitivity of the echogenicity, which because of its reversibility may have the future potential of deriving pressure curves from contrast images.

SH U 454 is the first ultrasonic contrast agent approved by health authorities. Together with its transpulmonary derivative SH U 508 A it is expected to extend the capability of diagnostic B-mode and Doppler ultrasound in a similarly dramatic way as the introduction of X-ray and magnetic resonance imaging contrast media did in their respective fields.

References

1. Gramiak R, Shah PM (1968) Echoacardiography of the aortic root. Invest Radiol 3: 356
2. Meltzer RS, Tickner G, Sahines TP, Popp RL (1980) The source of ultrasound contrast effect. J Clin Ultrasound 8: 121
3. Ophir J, Parker KJ (1989) Contrast agents in diagnostic ultrasound. Ultrasound Med Biol 15/4: 319–333
4. Schlief R (1991) Ultrasound contrast agents. Curr Opin Radiol 3: 198–207
5. Mottley J, Everbach EC, Schwarz KO et al. (1990) Decay of ultrasound integrated backscatter from a saccharide contrast agent is accelerated by increased pressure. Circulation 82/4 [Suppl III]: 28
6. Schlief R, Cramer E, Poland H (1990) Echokardiographische Druckmessungen mit Ultraschall-Kontrastmitteln? Z Kardiol 79 [Suppl I]: 17 (abstr)
7. Williams AR, Kubowicz G, Cramer E, Schlief R (1991) The effects of the microbubble suspension SH U 454 (Echovist) on ultrasound-induced cell lysis in a rotating tube exposure system. Echocardiography 8 (4): 423–433
8. Schlief R, Deichert U (1991) Hysterosalpingo-contrast sonography of the uterus and fallopian tubes: results of a clinical trial of a new contrast medium in 120 patients. Radiology 178: 213–215
9. Schlief R (1988) Echovist: Physikalisch-pharmakologische Eigenschaften, Ergebnisse klinischer Prüfungen und Anwendungspotential eines neuartigen Ultraschall-Kontrastmittels. In: Jahrbuch der Radiologie. Regensberg and Biermann, Münster, pp 163–170
10. Schlief R, Staks T, Mahler M et al. (1990) Successful opacification of the left heart chambers on echocardiographic examination after intravenous injection of a new saccharide based contrast agent. Echocardiography 7: 61–64
11. Becher H, von Bibra H, Glänzer K, Schlief R, Aupperle B, Vetter H (1990) Contrast enhanced doppler imaging of left heart chambers – first clinical results. Circulation 82/4 [Suppl III]: 95

Ultrasound Backscatter of Liver with Particulate Contrast Agents

T. A. Tuthill, R. B. Baggs, M. R. Violante, and K. J. Parker

Introduction

A solid-particle contrast agent in liver has provided some encouraging initial results [7, 8]. Iodipamide ethyl ester (IDE) can be formulated with a narrow diameter distribution about a mean which can be selected within the range of 0.1–2.0 μm. The particles can be prepared under sterile conditions, are stable over time, and do not clump in the blood after intravenous injection. The circulating particles are then captured by the Kupffer's cells which line the sinusoids of normal liver, and the IDE is eliminated within 2 days. The high density (2.4 g/cm^3) of these particles compared to surrounding tissue (1.0–1.1 g/cm^3) produces an impedance mismatch which is responsible for backscatter enhancement. Since tumors and other lesions lack Kupffer's cells, they do not concentrate the particles and therefore lack contrast effects compared to surrounding normal tissue. In previous work we have reported some of the ultrasonic properties ex vivo of liver with IDE [7], and imaging results in vivo of rabbit liver implanted with VX2 carcinomas [8]. This paper describes the measurement of ultrasonic backscatter in rabbit liver with standard IDE particles and with a newly formulated bubble-IDE particle. The changes in backscatter due to IDE uptake are related to those predicted by simple theory. The influence of biodistribution is examined. The results elucidate some of the underlying mechanisms of ultrasound propagation through normal liver and also underscore the importance of biodistribution in determining the ultrasonic effects of contrast agents.

Theory

For solid particles, the theoretical backscatter can be determined from the long wavelength approximation for scattering from an inhomogeneity of compressibility ($\varkappa_s$) and density (ϱ_s) in a fluid medium. The scattering cross-section (σ) is then a function of the difference in material properties. It is also proportional to the frequency to the fourth power and to the scatterer radius *(a)* to the sixth power. When a "cloud" of randomly positioned scatterers of concentration *(N)* per unit volume is present, the scattering cross-section, which is proportional to the total scattered power, simply increases with the concentration [4]:

$$\sigma = N\frac{4\pi}{9}\, k^4a^6 \left\{ \left| \frac{\varkappa_s - \varkappa}{\varkappa} \right|^2 + \frac{1}{3} \left| \frac{3(\varrho_s - \varrho)}{2\varrho_s + \varrho} \right|^2 \right\} \tag{1}$$

where k is the wavenumber, which is proportional to frequency and inversely proportional to wavelength. In the long wavelength approximation, the scatterer is assumed to be small, i.e., $ka << 1$. A general discussion of this equation with respect to contrast agents is given by Ophir and Parker [6]. In the current study we examine the effects of dose and also of particle size at constant dose, as predicted by Eq. 1. The concentration of a substance in an organ is one of the primary variables in toxicity considerations. The concentration (D, grams of contrast agent per cubic millimeter of tissue) is related to the conventional variables as:

$$D = N\left(\frac{4\pi}{3}\, a^3\right)\varrho_s \tag{2}$$

and so we rewrite the scattering equation as

$$\sigma = \left(\frac{1}{3\varrho_s}\right) Dk^4a^3\ \{\Delta z^2\} \tag{3}$$

where Δz represents the compressibility and density terms in brackets in Eq. 1. This theoretical representation shows that scattered power increases linearly with increased dose or concentration. Also, if the total dose is held constant while particle radius is increased, the scattered power increases only as the cube of radius, not the sixth power as is commonly inferred from Eq. 1. Assuming that the directionality of the scattering is independent of size in this long wavelength approximation, then for a constant dose, the root mean square (RMS) amplitude of a backscattered echo increases with radius to the 3/2 power, a relatively modest increase.

Methods

IDE and Rabbit Liver Preparations. The preparation for the solid, dense IDE particles has been described elsewhere [7]. For the in vitro studies, the particles were suspended in a bovine plasma distilled water (1 : 1) solution and placed in a small plastic pipette. In the animal studies, New Zealand white rabbits (Hazelton Laboratories), weighing 2–4 kg, were anesthetized and injected intravenously with a 10- to 15-ml (depending on weight) IDE suspension (final concentration of approximately 100 mg/ml) at a rate of 1 ml/min. The rabbits were scanned periodically using a clinical scanner. At 2 h some of the rabbits were sacrificed with a pentobarbital overdose and their livers excised immediately and placed in chilled, degassed saline. During measurements the livers were packed in a pill-box container, massaged to remove air bubbles, and secured by taut plastic wrap covers on the top and bottom, thereby providing flat surfaces. All ultrasound measurements were made at room temperature and within 3 h of excision.

Backscatter. A pulse-echo technique was used to determine relative backscatter. A wideband, 10 MHz center frequency, Panametrics transducer (1.3 cm diameter, 5 cm focus), driven by a JSR Pulser, was used to obtain RF scan lines. For the in vitro measurements the mean backscatter (RMS) was computed for three uncorrelated scan lines, each corresponding to 4 mm in length. In the ex vivo studies, eight scan lines were taken from the anterior region of the right medial lobe. The stored data corresponded to 4 mm of tissue, starting at 1 mm below the surface to avoid ring-down effects. Precaution against specular reflectors was taken by monitoring the signal-to-noise ratio (SNR) and saving scan lines only where the SNR was greater than 1.5 [II]. A standard deviation of 18 % for the SNR is expected based on the properties of speckle.

Water Content. To measure water content three pieces (≈0.5 g) were taken from each liver, cut into smaller pieces, and placed in glass containers to be weighed. The three samples were then heated at 90 °C in a vacuum for 16 h, cooled in a desiccator, and reweighed. The weight loss then determines the water content. The accuracy is estimated as less than 1 %.

Results

The Normal Rabbit Liver. The raw backscatter echo amplitude from 16 normal livers ranged from 0.12 to 0.18 mV RMS with an average of 0.15 mV (67 dB below the RMS echo from a perfect reflector). This large variation in normal values was found to depend partly on variations in the wet to dry weights of the liver specimens, as shown in Fig. 1. The solid line is a theoretical curve obtained by assuming that the backscatter (intensity) is linearly proportional to the solid weight of the liver, with zero backscatter at zero solid weight. The dependence of backscatter on water weight was noted by Bamber et al. [1].

The Normal Liver with Standard IDE. Data for liver with IDE, under experimental conditions covering a wide range of doses and particle sizes, are also shown in Fig. 1. The backscatter amplitudes are plotted as a function of water percentage to demonstrate that the average water content of IDE liver (mean value 72.1 % ± 1.4 %) is similar to that of control liver (mean value 72.0 % ± 1.0 %). This implies that no significant inflammatory reaction is initiated by the IDE, and thus that any change in backscatter is due to the presence of the particles themselves, not to any change in the organ.

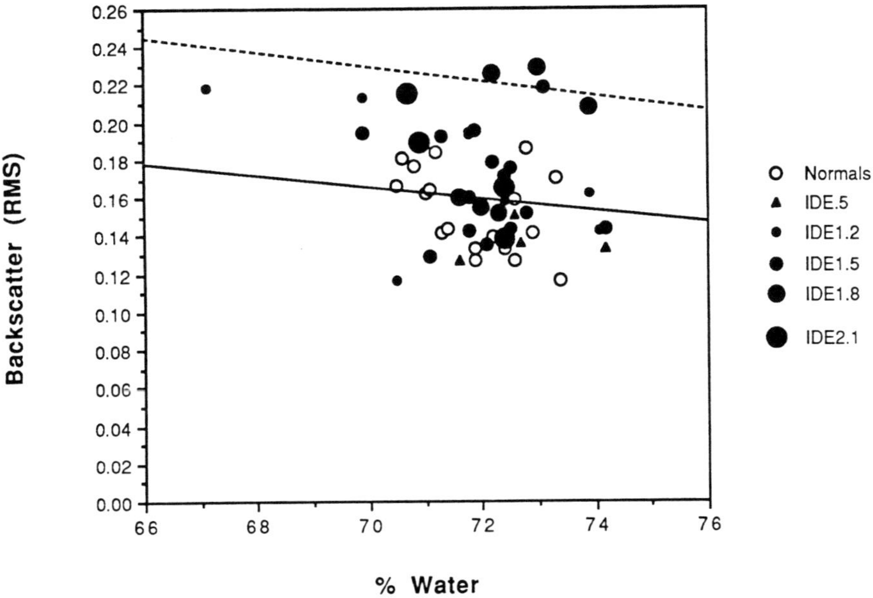

Fig. 1. Raw backscatter values (RMS) of all measured livers plotted versus water content. *Open circles,* normal livers; *solid symbols,* IDE livers for a range of doses and particle sizes. *Solid line* is from theory assuming that the backscatter intensity is proportional to solid weight; *dotted line* is 3 dB above the solid line, representing a desireable increase in backscatter for lesion detection in speckle

Biodistribution. Within the past decade some reports have indicated that the concentration of Kupffer's cells is heterogeneous, the highest concentration being in the periportal region [9]. In addition, the periportal Kupffer's cells have a higher endocytic activity. Our histology sections of IDE liver support this; a marked concentration of particles is observed within selected Kupffer's cells that lie near the outflow of the portal triads, in a pattern which can be termed a peripheral lobular distribution. Examination by scanning electron microscopy shows that Kupffer's cells capture up to 30 particles [2]. Thus, a concentration of scatterers occurs at two levels. At the level of the Kupffer's cells (scale approximately 10 μm) IDE is captured and held in groups of up to 30 particles. At the lobular level (scale approximately 1 mm), the IDE-bearing Kupffer's cells are concentrated in a peripheral lobular distribution. This pattern was observed over a range of doses (100–600 mg IDE/kg body weight) and particle sizes (1.2–2.1 μm diameter) in experiments in normal rabbit liver.

Bubble-IDE Particles. A new formulation of IDE introduces gas into the manufacturing process such that the gas is stabilized on the micron-sized particles. These bubble-IDE particles show a marked increase in echogenicity over standard IDE preparations. Fig. 2 shows the RMS values of in vitro

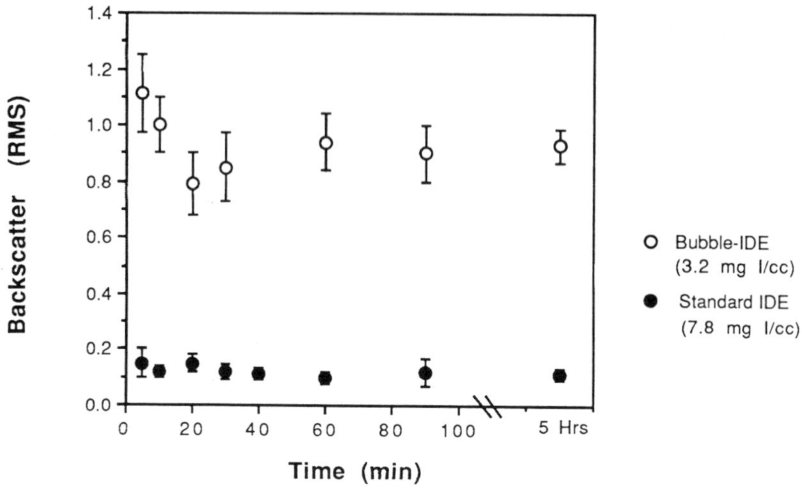

Fig. 2. Raw backscatter values (RMS) of in vitro particle solutions, bubble-IDE (3.2 mg I/cm^3) and standard IDE (7.8 mg I/cm^3), plotted versus time

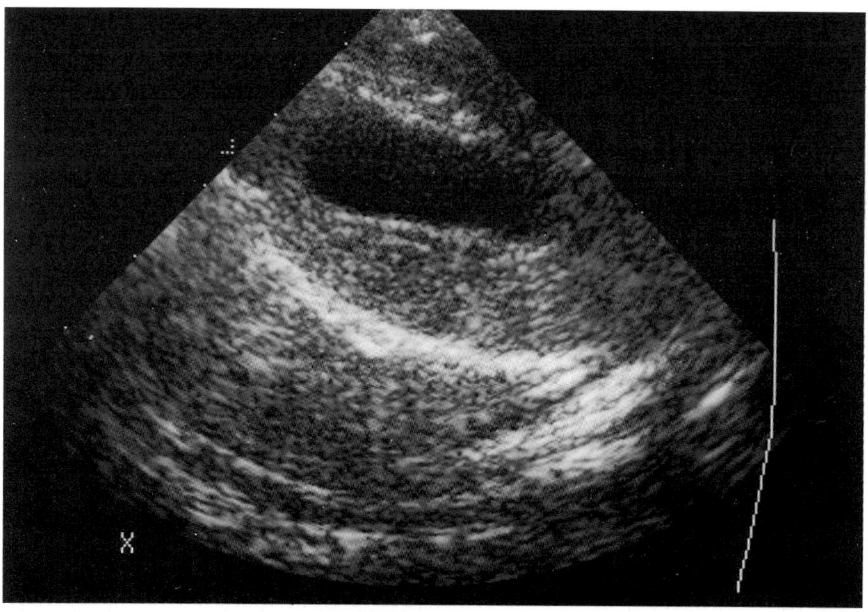

Fig. 3. B-scan image at 5 MHz of normal rabbit liver with gall bladder before infusion of the bubble-IDE contrast agent

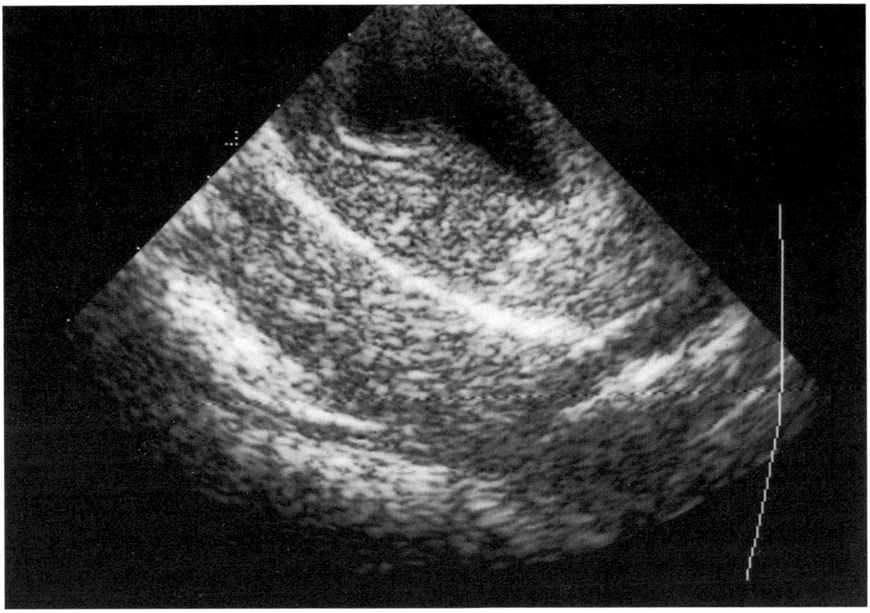

Fig. 4. Same liver as in Fig. 3 and same constant gain settings, but 60 min following intravenous infusion of the bubble/particle agent. Note the enhancement of the parenchymal echogenicity, which was observed until approximately 120 min

particle solutions versus time, demonstrating the particles' stability. Note that the concentration of the bubble-IDE solution is less than half that of the standard IDE. B-scan images of rabbit liver with and without the bubble-IDE particles are shown in Figs. 3 and 4. These images were obtained from a 5.0-MHz Acuson scanner with all settings held absolutely constant over a 120-min examination period. The injected dose of the bubble-IDE agent was approximately 200 mg IDE/kg body weight, and direct visualization of the agent in the right and left heart chambers and the portal vein was possible at 0–10 min from the start of the injection due to the increased echogenicity of this agent.

Discussion and Conclusion

The normal rabbit liver properties are influenced by water content. The backscatter data show a trend towards decreasing echogenicity with increasing water content, as noted by Bamber et al. [1]. When IDE is added, there is no change in average water content. The resulting increase in backscatter depends on the particle size and dose administered and can be approximately a 3-dB increase in echo strength for 1.2-μm particles at 200–300 mg IDE/kg body weight. An increase of 3 dB is comparable to other backscatter variations which have been utilized in tissue characterization such as those associated with myocardial tissue [5]. Furthermore, 3 dB is a significant enhancement in regards to the lesion detection problem for fully developed speckle [3, 10]. This enhancement may be increased further by changing the density and compressibility properties of IDE in future research.

It must be emphasized that the backscatter does not follow the simple superposition of normal liver plus the addition of randomly positioned single particles of IDE. There is not, as theory predicts, a strong dependence on particle size. There is not, as theory predicts, a monotonic increase with dose. Furthermore, the overall increase is larger than would be expected from preliminary in vitro studies of IDE suspensions in gelatin, which would predict a 1 dB increase for 1.2-μm particles at a final concentration of 5 mg IDE/cm^3, instead of the 3 dB observed.

Presumably, the explanation for these gross discrepancies lies with the concentration effects by the Kupffer's cells in the peripheral lobular regions. The effect of this biodistribution on scattering is not known theoretically but is addressed using mathematical models and the optical staining – transform methods of [12].

Also, the accumulation of IDE particles in the presence of a tumor needs to be examined. Kupffer's cells are known to surround tumor cells in their early stages [13], although as the tumor grows, this process is blocked by tumor cell products. This initial encirclement may produce a ring of IDE particles and further enhance the contrast between tumor and healthy tissue.

The mechanisms which produce a distinct peripheral lobular distribution of particles are not fully understood and require further research. Presumably the pattern of particle acquisition is germane to other classes of dense, solid particles which may be formulated for X-ray or magnetic resonance imaging enhancement. Thus, the biodistribution effects may prove important to other imaging modalities in addition to ultrasound.

When gas is stabilized on modified IDE particles, the resulting particle – bubble agent has high echogenicity compared to IDE and has long stability in vitro and in vivo. Preliminary results in rabbits demonstrate the possibility that the stabilized, echogenic gas can be delivered to the Kupffer's cells of the liver, raising the backscatter well above the levels obtained with standard IDE. Because IDE is also useful as a computed tomography agent, this compound may have wide utility as a multimodality agent.

Acknowledgement. This work was supported by NIH grant no. CA44732. We are grateful for the expert experimental assistance of Mr. P. Dentinger and Ms. D. Hartley.

References

1. Bamber JC, Hill CR, King JA (1981) Acoustic properties of normal and cancerous human liver. II. Dependence on tissue structure. Ultrasound Med Biol 7: 135–144
2. Lauteala L, Komano M, Violante M (1984) Effect of IV administered IDE particles on rat liver morphology. Invest Radiol 19: 133–141
3. Lowe H, Bamber JC, Webb S, Cook-Martin G (1988) Perceptual studies of contrast, texture, and detail in ultrasound B-scans. SPIE Med Imaging II 914: 40–47
4. Morse PM, Ingard KU (1968) Theoretical acoustics. McGraw-Hill, New York, p 427
5. Mottley JG, Miller JG (1988) Anisotropy of ultrasound backscatter of myocardial tissue. I. Theory and measurements in vitro. J Acoust Soc Am 83: 755–761
6. Ophir J, Parker KJ (1989) Contrast agents in diagnostic ultrasound. Ultrasound Med Biol 15: 319–333
7. Parker KJ, Tuthill TA, Lerner RM, Violante MR (1987) A particulate contrast agent with potential for ultrasound imaging of liver. Ultrasound Med Biol 13: 555–566
8. Parker KJ, Baggs RB, Lerner RM, Tuthill TA, Violante MR (1990) Ultrasound contrast for hepatic tumors using IDE particles. Invest Radiol 25: 1135–1139
9. Sleyster EC, Knook DL (1982) Relation between localization and function of rat liver Kupffer cells. Lab Invest 47: 484–490
10. Sperry RH, Parker KJ (1991) Segmentation of speckle images based on level crossing statistics. J Opt Soc Am [A] 8 (3): 490–498
11. Tuthill TA, Sperry RH, Parker KJ (1988) Deviations from Rayleigh statistics in ultrasonic speckle. Ultrason Imaging 10: 81–89
12. Waag RC, Nilsson JO, Astheimer JP (1983) Characterization of volume scattering power spectra in isotropic media from power spectra of scattering by planes. J Acoust Soc Am 74: 1555–1571
13. Wake K, Decker K, Kirn A, Knook DL, McCuskey RS, Bouwens L, Wisse E (1989) Cell biology and kinetics of Kupffer cells in the liver. Int Rev Cytol 118: 173–229

Diagnosis of Colon Tumors and Inflammatory Large-Bowel Diseases by Hydro-colonic Sonography

B. Limberg

Introduction

Abdominal sonography has proven to be of great value in evaluating many abdominal diseases and has over the years become an accepted and effective primary imaging modality. However, conventional abdominal sonography does have its limitations when used in assessing the gastrointestinal tract. Due to the presence of luminal gas within the bowel, which limits a full and detailed evaluation of the bowel wall and bowel lumen, the interpretation of diseases of the bowel tend to be both difficult and inexact. Conventional sonography has therefore played only a subordinate role as a diagnostic procedure for the diagnosis of colon tumors and inflammatory large bowel diseases [1, 2].

Normal bowel loops have an amorphous appearance, but experience has shown that whenever an ileus is present, the additional intraluminal fluid improves sonographic visibility and allows for a more complete examination of the bowel. In this situation under optimal conditions the serrated pattern of the valvulae conniventes and the thickness of the intestinal wall can be observed [3].

It therefore appeared worthwhile to investigate whether hydro-colonic sonography (the retrograde instillation of fluid into the colon prior to sonographic examination) would similarly improve the clarity of sonographic images and prove to be of diagnostic value in evaluating various diseases of the colon.

Method

Optimal preparation and the use of a high-frequency transducer are the two essentials for performing hydro-colonic sonography. Bowel preparation consists of a laxative orthograde intestinal lavage on the morning of examination. A total of up to 1500 ml water can be instilled retrogradely into the colon after intravenous injection of 20 mg *n*-butyl-scopolamine bromide (Buscopan, Boehringer Ingelheim). The relaxant is not only a necessity to achieve optimal distension of the bowel during water instillation but also serves to suppress the sense of urgency for bowel elimination, which enables even older patients to hold the instilled water easily. Continuous transabdominal sonographic examination of the large intestine, beginning at the time of water instillation, is carried out using a real-time scanning device with a 3.5-, 5.0-, and 7.5-MHz transducer (Picker CS 9500).

The examination is started using the 3.5-MHz transducer to obtain an overview. For more detailed examination the 5.0- and the 7.5-MHz transducers are then used. A manual tilting table is recommended. When sonography begins, the patient should be oblique to achieve distension of the rectosigmoid transition and the sigmoid. Water (300–500 ml) is then instilled. The descending, transverse, and ascending colon are then examined with the patient supine, with a further 900–1000 ml being instilled. The examination lasts approximately 15 min. Hydro-colonic sonography is not perceived by patients to be uncomfortable, and the method has a high acceptance rate.

The diagnosis of colonic tumors is based on finding evidence of intraluminal masses fixed to the wall or lesions within the intestinal wall structure and/or in the surrounding connective tissue.

For the diagnosis of inflammatory large-bowel diseases important indications include alterations of bowel wall echogenicity, a thickening of the bowel wall and evidence of abnormalities in the bowel wall layers.

Hydro-colonic Sonography of the Normal Colon

The results of our studies show that with the retrograde instillation of water the entire length of the colon, starting at the rectosigmoid junction and ending at the cecum, can be visualized sonographically in 97 % of cases [4, 5]. The rectum, however, cannot be visualized in detail due to overlying air and the penetration limits of the transducers. In some patients total evaluation of the colon is not possible because of the presence of feces or of air in the bowel lumen or because of a elongated sigmoid or transverse colon. The sonographic images obtained from healthy subjects using this technique show an echo-free intestinal lumen with a width of 4–5 cm, with the haustra projecting as echogenic indentations into the lumen (Figs. 1, 2). The Bauhin's valve is seen as an echogenic polypoid lesion projecting into the lumen (Fig. 3). After the instilled water reaches the ileum, the junction of the cecum with the ileum can be visualized. Using a high-frequencey transducer it is possible not only to judge the haustra and the width of the intestinal lumen but also to view in detail the bowel wall structure. Five layers of different echogenicity can be distinguished within the bowel wall (Fig. 4). Along the margin of the lumen a thin, echogenic layer can be seen. Going deeper, there is a thin, echo-poor layer, followed by a thicker, echogenic layer then a thicker, echo-poor layer, and finally an outer echogenic layer. The total width of the intestinal wall is 3–4 mm. The sonographically demonstrable layers correspond to the anatomic layers of the colon wall. The mucosa is represented by the first two layers; the submucosa corresponds to the third echogenic layer; the muscularis propria to the fourth, echo-poor layer; and the subserosal fat and the subserosa to the fifth, echogenic layer [6]. The sonographic images of the

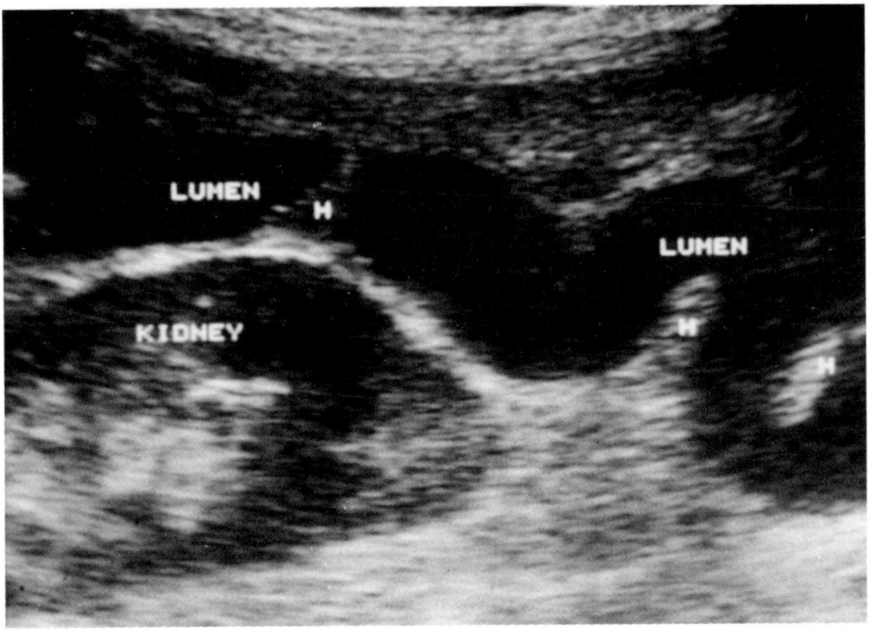

Fig. 1. Normal colon. The fluid-filled lumen appears as an echo-free ribbon-shaped structure. The haustra *(H)* project as echogenic indentations into the lumen

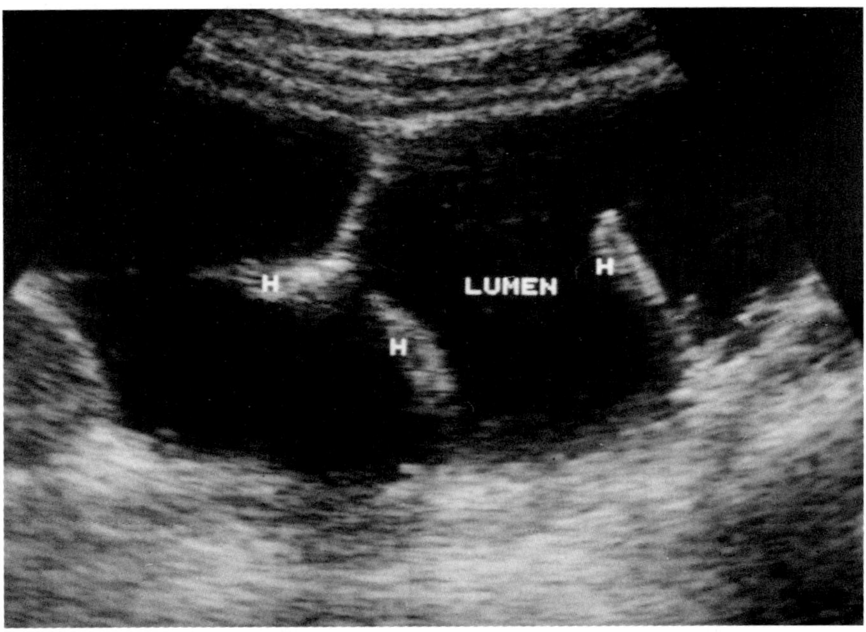

Fig. 2. Normal colon. Enlarged portion of the ascending colon with typical haustration *(H)*

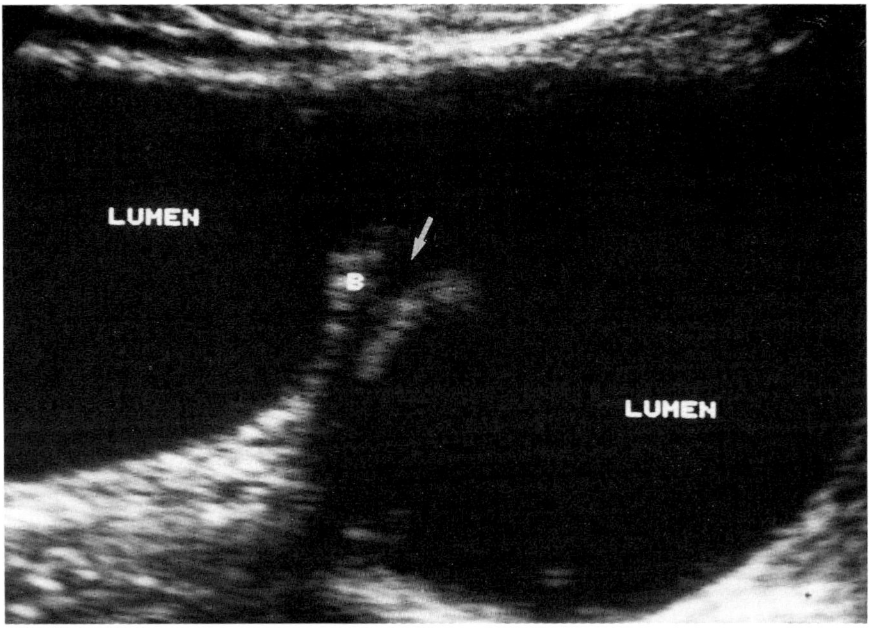

Fig. 3. Normal fluid-filled cecum with Bauhin's valve *(B)* that projects as a polypoid lesion into the lumen. The orifice of the Bauhin's valve is clearly visible *(arrow)*

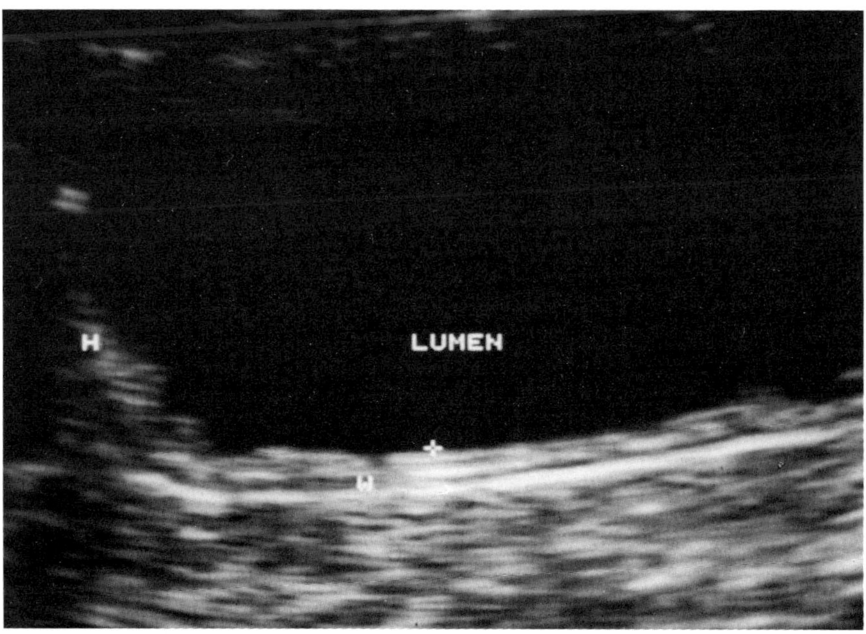

Fig. 4. Normal colon, enlarged portion of the gastrointestinal wall. Within the colon wall *(W)* five individual layers can be demonstrated. Beginning luminally: a thin echogenic layer, then a thin echo-poor, followed by a thicker echogenic, and again an echo-poor layer, finally the outer boundary – an echogenic layer

colon wall displayed during hydro-colonic sonography correspond with the images obtained during endorectal sonography and by endosonography of the upper gastrointestinal tract [7, 8].

Hydro-colonic Sonography of Colon Tumors

Colonic polyps and carcinomas appear sonographically as echogenic structures projecting from the intestinal wall into the lumen [5]. Pedunculated polyps float in the lumen whenever the abdomen is compressed or the patient's position changes. During sonography the peduncle of the polyp and the head of the polyp can be clearly seen, and pedunculated polyps can easily be differentiated from sessile polyps (Fig. 5). At the base of the polyp the typical wall structure remains and can be identified by hydro-colonic sonography. Whenever no visible destruction or alteration in the echogenicity of the colon wall is discernible, it can be assumed that there is no infiltration into the wall (Figs. 6, 7). The statistically determined sensitivity for the detection of polyps larger than 7 mm is 91%. Small polyps (<7 mm) cannot always be demonstrated. The diagnosis of small polyps is difficult because they cannot always be differentiated from nearby haustra.

Colonic carcinomas appear sonographically as echogenic structures that project into the intestinal lumen and are fixed to the colon wall. Favorable

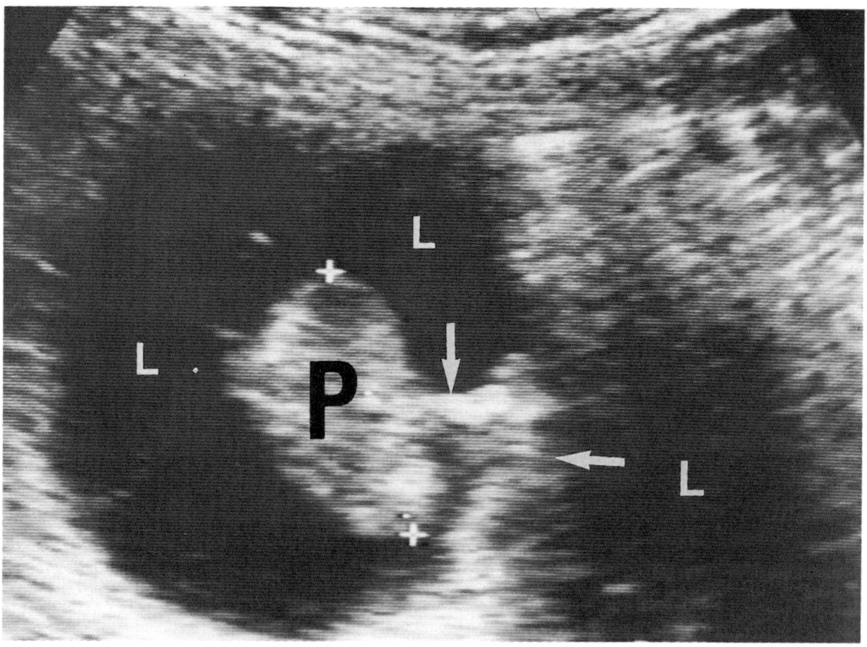

Fig. 5. Pedunculated polyp projecting as an echogenic tumor into the colon lumen *(L)*. The head *(P)* of the polyp can be clearly seen; *arrows* pinpoint the peduncle

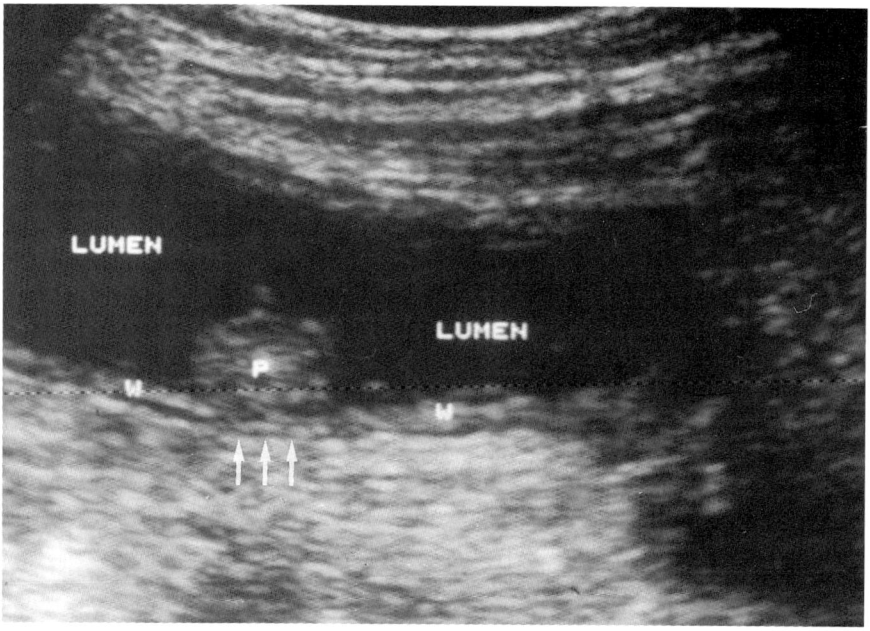

Fig. 6. Small colonic polyp *(P)*. The tumor is fixed to the bowel wall. At the base of the polyp the typical five-layer structure of the colon wall *(W)* remains *(arrows)*

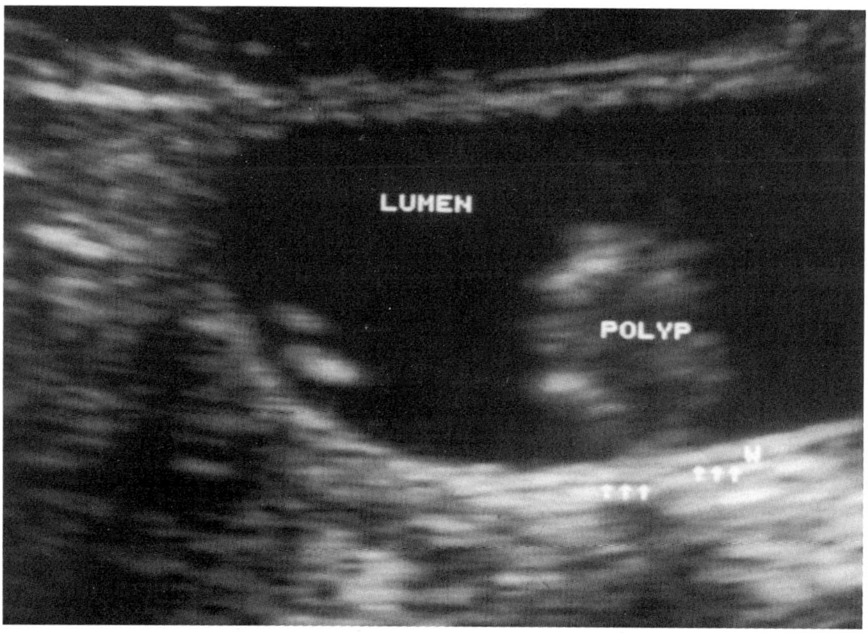

Fig. 7. Polyp with a very small peduncle. The wall structure *(arrows)* at the base of the polyp is intact

examination conditions also allow for the sonographic demonstration of wall infiltration (Figs. 8, 9). In most cases the image projected by the infiltrating tumor is less echogenic than the submucosa and the surrounding connective tissue. The extent of invasion can be evaluated by observing the irregularities in the bowel layer structure. By using hydro-colonic sonography a more exact staging of the tumors according to the TNM classification of the International Union Against Cancer is possible [9]. The T aspect can be assessed by hydro-colonic sonography using the following criteria: T1, the tumor disturbs the first two layers, i.e., it is confined to the mucosa; T2, the tumor disturbs layers 1–3, i.e., it infiltrates the submucosa; T3, the tumor disturbs layers 1–5, i.e., it infiltrates the colon wall and the surrounding connective tissue; T4, the tumor is such that all bowel wall layers are disturbed and other organs are infiltrated as well.

Our results show that using hydro-colonic sonography made it possible to correctly determine the T stage of colon carcinomas in 82 % of cases. Because there were no T1 carcinomas in our study, it is not possible at present to say conclusively whether hydro-colonic sonography enables a differentiation of benign polyps and T1 carcinomas with infiltration limited to the mucosa and submucosa.

Colon tumors can be confused with stool particles, which also appear as echogenic structures within the bowel lumen. In contrast to colon tumors, however, stool particles are most often accompanied by an acoustic shadow, probably caused from colonic gas within the stool particles (Fig. 10). Using

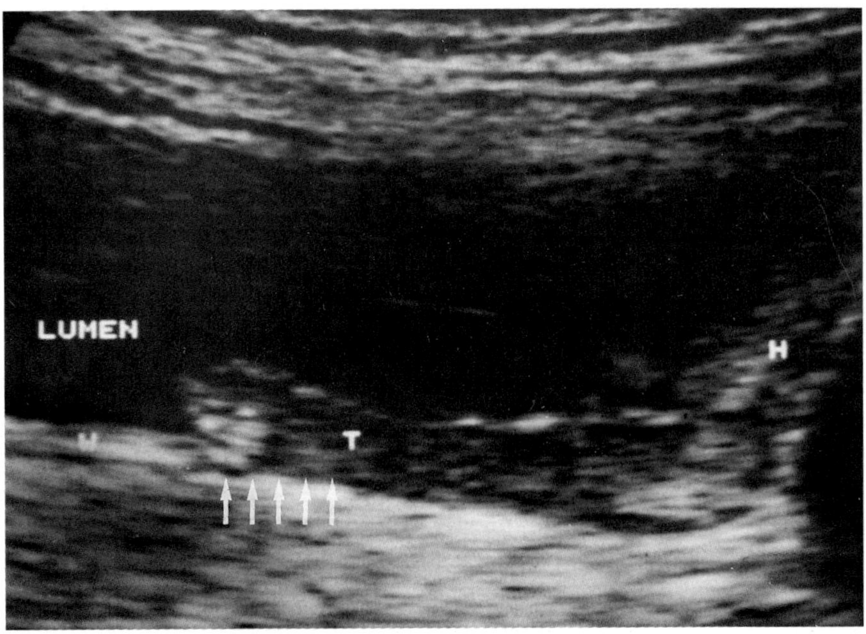

Fig. 8. Colonic carcinoma *(T)*. The depth of tumor infiltration is confined to the muscularis propria *(arrows)*. *W*, Colon wall; *H*, haustra

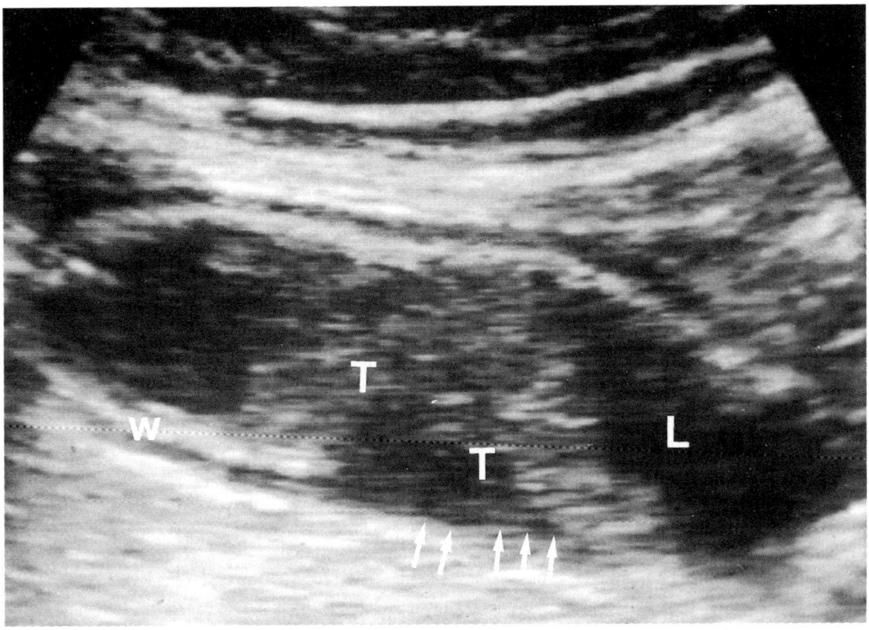

Fig. 9. Colonic carcinoma. All layers are disturbed, and the tumor infiltrates the surrounding tissue *(arrows)*

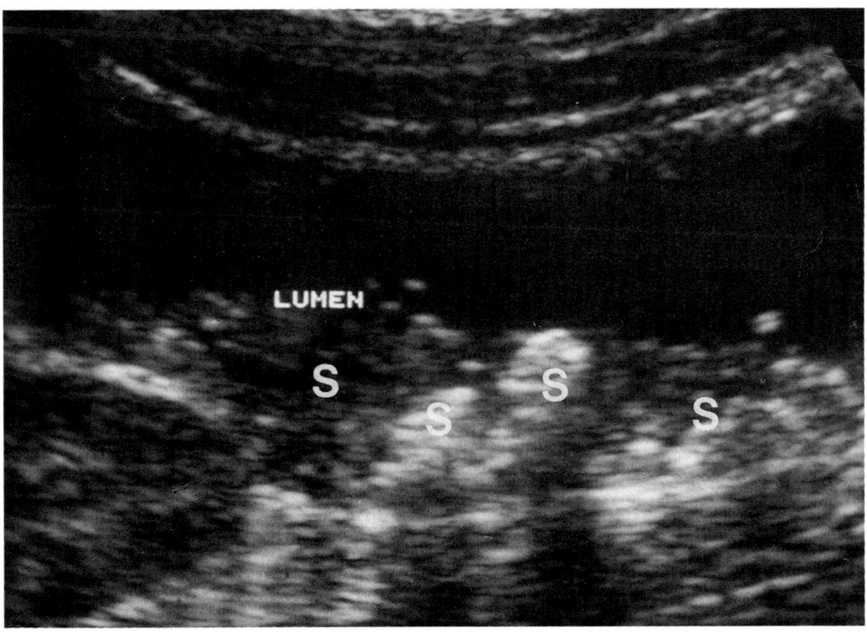

Fig. 10. Stool particles. The stool particles *(S)* appear as echogenic, mobile structures often accompanied by an acoustic shadow

real-time equipment makes it possible to observe peristalsis of the fluid-filled bowel as well as movement of particulate material or gas bubbles within the colon lumen. A quick light compression with the transducer on the abdomen may induce peristalsis and cause stool particles or gas bubbles to move, thereby allowing a clear differentiation between artifacts and real pathologic alterations of the large bowel wall.

Hydro-colonic Sonography in Inflammatory Large-Bowel Diseases

Hydro-colonic sonography makes it possible to demonstrate not only neoplastic diseases of the colon but also acute inflammatory large bowel diseases, for example, active Crohn's disease and ulcerative colitis [4, 10, 11]. Sonographic examination of the gastrointestinal wall layers is important for the diagnosis and differential diagnosis of these diseases. In most patients with Crohn's disease, the normal five-layer structure of the colonic wall is no longer in evidence, and the wall becomes echo-poor and increases in thickness (up to 1.5 cm; Fig. 11). However, in those patients whose Crohn's disease is coupled only with aphthous ulcerations the wall becomes echo-poor, but the typical wall stratification remains intact, suggesting that the

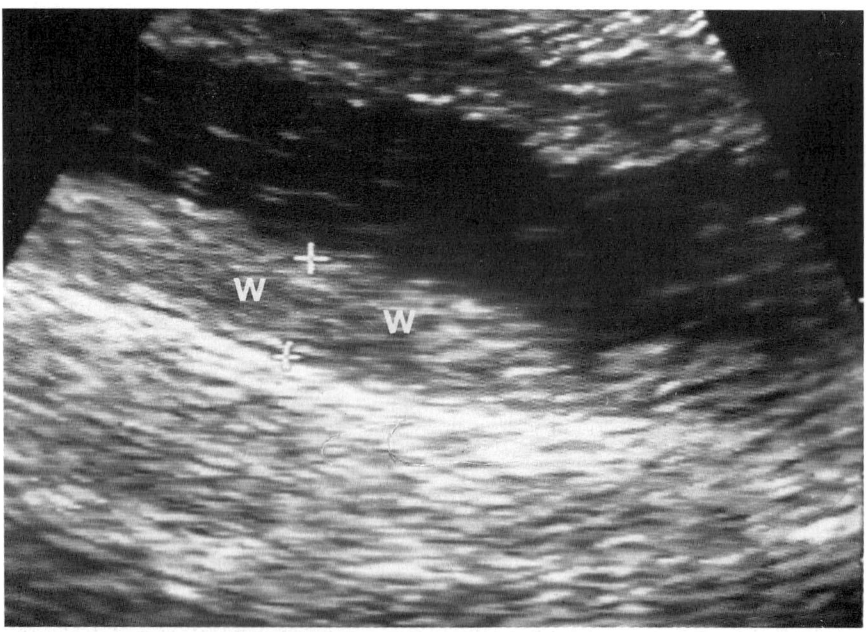

Fig. 11. Acute Crohn's disease of the colon. The colon wall *(W)* is clearly thickened and appears echo-poor. The typical five-layer structure of the colon wall and the haustra are no longer demonstrable

structural alterations are superficial rather than transmural. It is only as the inflammation becomes transmural that the five-layer stratification of the colon wall can no longer be recognized. Typically, a differentiation between layers 1, 2, and 3 is no longer possible, and layers 4 and 5 are seen only rudimentarily. Finally, in advanced stages of Crohn's disease a visualization of the wall stratification is no longer possible and the wall appears homogeneous. In active ulcerative colitis the colonic wall also becomes echo-poor, but its thickness is only moderately increased, and the five-layer structure is still clearly in evidence (Fig. 12). When ulcerative colitis is accompanied by extensive inflammatory pseudopolyposis however, the five layers are no longer so easily discernible so that a clear differentiation from Crohn's disease becomes difficult. In such cases the sonographic detection of extensive inflammatory pseudopolyposis helps in making the diagnosis of ulcerative colitis. Crohn's disease could be differentiated from ulcerative colitis in 86 % of the cases when hydro-colonic sonography was used.

Our study indicates that hydro-colonic sonography enables a detailed sonographic examination of the colon lumen and the colon wall, thus providing additional information for a more exact diagnosis of many diseases of the colon.

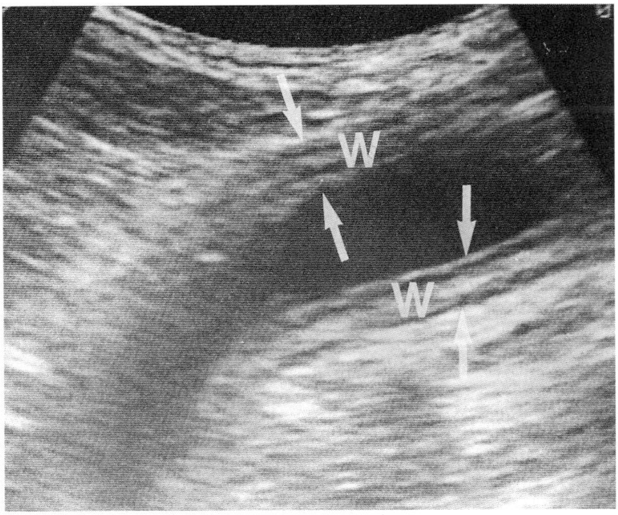

Fig. 12. Acute ulcerative colitis of the colon. The colon wall *(W)* appears echo-poor and is only moderately thickened. The typical wall stratification of five layers *(arrows)* remains. The quality with which hydro-colonic sonography reveals the first two layers representing the mucosa is remarkable

References

1. Lutz HT, Petzold R (1976) Ultrasonographic patterns of space occupying lesions of the stomach and the intestine. Ultrasound Med Biol 2: 129–132
2. Bluth EI, Merritt CRB, Sullivan MA (1979) Ultrasonic evaluation of the stomach, small bowel, and colon. Radiology 133: 677–680
3. Limberg B (1988) Diagnosis of inflammatory and neoplastic large bowel diseases by conventional abdominal and colonic sonography. Ultrasound Q 6: 151–166
4. Limberg B (1989) Diagnosis of acute ulcerative colitis and colonic Crohn's disease by colonic sonography. J Clin Ultrasound 17: 25–31
5. Limberg B (1990) Diagnosis of large bowel tumours by colonic sonography. Lancet 335: 144–146
6. Kimmey MB, Martin RW, Haggitt RC, Wand KY, Franklin DW, Silverstein FE (1989) Histologic correlates of gastrointestinal ultrasound images. Gastroenterology 96: 433–441
7. Hildebrandt U, Feifel G (1985) Preoperative staging of rectal cancer by intrarectal ultrasound. Dis Colon Rectum 28: 42–46
8. Tio TL, Cohen P, Coene PP, Udding J, Den Hartog Jager FCA, Tytgat GNJ (1989) Endosonography and computed tomography of esophageal carcinoma. Gastroenterology 96: 1478–1486
9. Hermanek P, Sobin LH (eds) (1987) TNM classification of malignant tumors, 4th edn. International Union Against Cancer. Springer, Berlin Heidelberg New York
10. Limberg B (1990) Sonographic features of colonic Crohn's disease – comparison of in vivo and in vitro studies. J Clin Ultrasound 18: 161–166
11. Limberg B (1990) Kolonsonographie – eine neue Methode zur Diagnostik von Morbus Crohn und Colitis ulcerosa. Monatsschr Kinderheilkd 138: 422–426

Endoscopic Ultrasound: Recent Advances in Gastroenterology

M. Fukuda, K. Hirata, M. Mitani, T. Mochizuki, and H. Tatuguchi

Until very recently, diagnostic approaches to diseases of the gastrointestinal (GI) tract were limited mostly to roentogenographic and endoscopic examinations. In routine practice these were performed in conjunction with appropriate biochemical studies. Endoscopy is an extremely effective procedure for evaluating mucosal lesions of the GI tract; however, these standard approaches have limitations in diseases involving the submucosal and extramural layers of the GI tract. Likewise, precise staging of carcinoma of the GI tract in terms of the depth of penetration is almost impossible. Diseases of organs adjacent to the GI tract, such as the pancreas, biliary tract, retroperitoneal spaces, infiltration of rectosigmoid cancer to the urinary bladder, parametrium, and female pelvic organs are extremely difficult to diagnose by these standard procedures. To overcome these limitations, endosonographic methods including sonoendoscopy has been developed.

History of Endoscopic Ultrasonosonography

Endoscopic ultrasound (EUS), endosonography conducted under optical guidance by endoscopic means, has been introduced relatively recently. However, the idea of endosonography for scanning intraabdominal organs, especially of the rectum, had been introduced as early as 1955 by Wild in Minneapolis USA. Two years later Wild and Reid [33] published an article on the use of transrectal scanner equipped with a 15-MHz transducer, by which the very first B-mode image of the rectal carcinoma was produced in vivo [34]. Because of this significant contribution in medical imaging, Wild was awarded the 1991 Japan Prize for biomedical imaging technology.

It took a considerable time, however, until EUS emerged even on an experimental basis. Preliminary reports on the use of EUS came from Japan and the United States [8, 16]. Interestingly, these investigators adopted entirely different scanning methods to obtain images by intraluminal scanning, the one with mechanical scanning and the other with an electronic scanning using a linear array transducer. Following these pioneering works, a number of commercial firms began manufacturing such instruments.

Equipment

After a series of prototype EUS equipments, Olympus (Tokyo, Japan) developed the first commercially available equipment, the GFUM1/EUM1 (Fig. 1). This equipment was aimed at the use of EUS for scanning of the upper GI tract. Subsequently, valuable diagnostic information was accumulated by EUS, especially on the staging of malignant neoplasms of the GI tract [4, 11, 15, 32], analysis of GI tract ulceration [2], examination of biliary, pancreatic diseases [6, 7, 9, 12, 14, 20, 21, 28, 29, 36], esophageal varices [5], and pathologic changes in the mediastinum [23, 25].

In the meantime a number of improvements were made in the system, especially as regards the sonoendoscope.

The requirements are the following [27]:

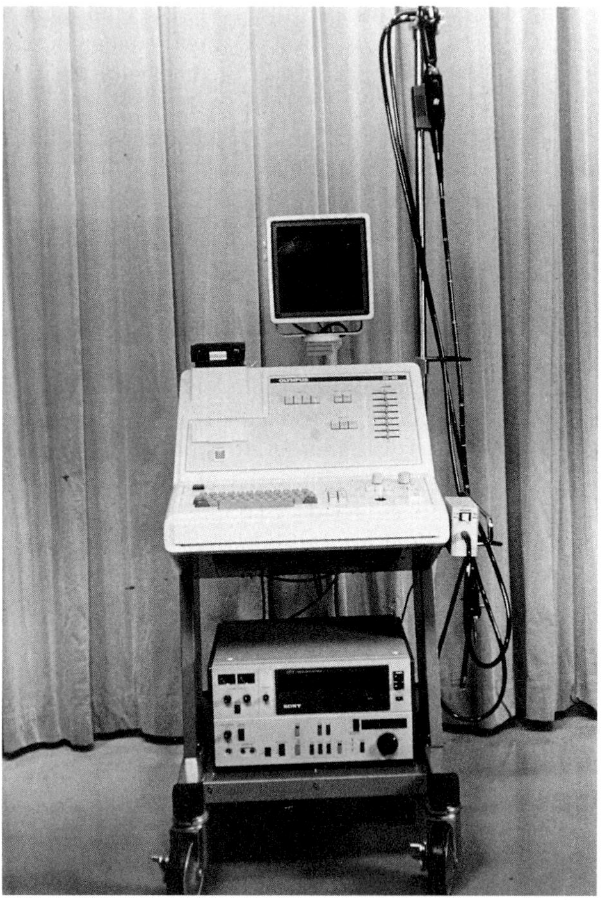

Fig. 1. Ultrasonic endoscope, Olympus GFUM1/EUM1. The first commercially available mechanical scanning sonoendoscope with the imaging unit, EUM1

1) addition of a biopsy channel,
2) switching of ultrasonic frequencies,
3) further compactness of the scan head and reduction in the weight and size of the manipulation section, and concentration of all the control switches to the scope to allow one-man operation, and
4) the use of higher frequencies. Furthermore, production of specific "scopes" according to the respective needs of examination was also advocated.

Other requirements included equipment for color Doppler presentation, image processing capabilities to the system, and combination with the videoendoscope. Within approximately 5 years after this proposal was made, most of these requirements were fulfilled.

Table 1 and Fig. 2 show an array of sonoendoscopes available in 1991. These are classified into two major groups, those with a radially scanning transducer and those with an electronic array transducer. The instruments in the former group are subdivided into scopes for the upper and those for the lower GI tracts. The sonocolonofiberscopes are thicker in diameter than other scopes because of the necessity to include an optical unit at the very front of the scope to facilitate safe insertion into the ascending colon via the tortuous

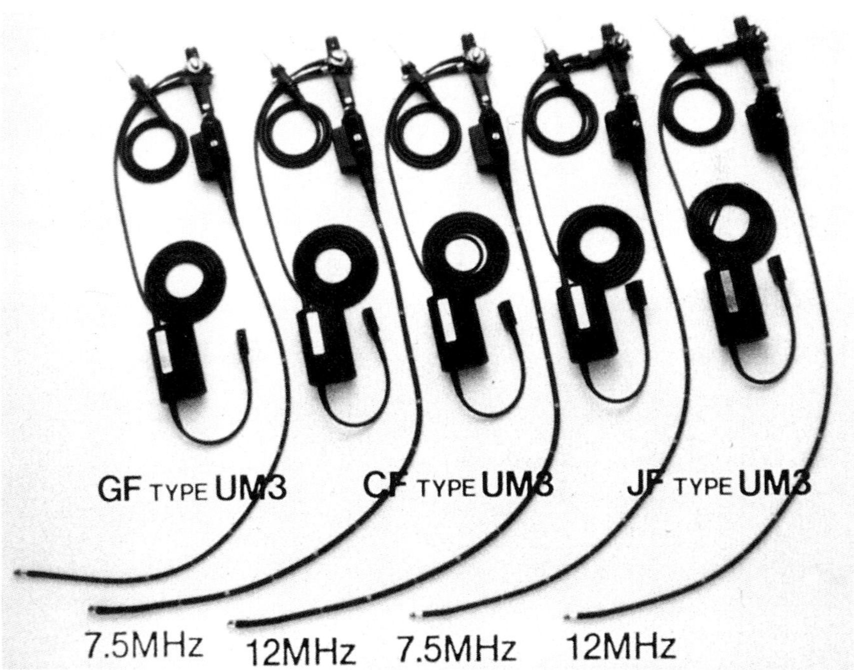

Fig. 2. An array of sonoendoscopes. Scopes for upper GI equipped with dual transducer system of 7.5 and 12 MHz (GFUM3), colonosonofiberscope (CFUM3), and scopes for transduodenal scanning (JFUM3)

Table 1. Commercially available EUS equipment

Manufacturer	Apparatus	Scanning mode	Transducer frequency (MHz)	Size	Application	Miscellaneous
Olympus	GFUM2/EUM2	360° radial	7.5/10	7 mm	Upper GI	Single disc
	GFUM3/EUM3	360° radial	7.5 + 12	7 mm	Upper GI	Dual disc
	JFUM3/EUM3	360° radial	7.5/12	7 mm	Duodenum	Single disc
	CFUM2/EUM2	360° radial	7.5/12	7 mm	Colon	Single disc
	CFUM3/EUM3	300° radial	7.5/12	7 mm	Colon	Single disc
	UM-1W/EUM3	360° radial	7.5	2 × 2 mm	GI	Single disc
	Convex Doppler		5/7.5	17 mm	GI	B-mode, Doppler
	LPS-US	Linear	7.5	25 mm	Laparoscope	B-mode
Toshiba	EPE/703FL	Linear	7.5	31 mm	GI	B-mode, Doppler
Pentax	FC 32 UA	Convex Doppler	5/7/5	30 mm	GI	B-mode, Doppler
Fujinon	SP101	Manual B-scan	20/15	2 × 2 mm	GI	B-mode
Diasonics		360° radial	20	1.35 mm		Radial scan

sigmoid (Fig. 3). In the Olympus JFUM sonoendoscope, specifically designed for transduodenal scanning, reduction in the size of scan-head compartment and increase in the flexion angle resulted in marked improvement in maneuvability of transduodenal scanning. In addition, the channel for a biopsy forceps or cannulation tube for endoscopic retrograde cholangiopancreatography (ERCP) were included (Fig. 4).

The electronic scanning sonoendoscope, on the other hand, has the disadvantage of a narrower view field compared to those with a mechanically rotating transducer, which give a complete 360° scan image. There are certain advantages over the latter in that the scope can use the ordinary ultrasound unit for imaging, thus adding such features as two-dimensional color flow Doppler from within the lumen of GI tract (Fig. 5). Scanning in the longitudinal directions and lesser grade of attenuation of ultrasound by the linear or convex arrays are the other merits of the method.

The latest topic in endosonography is the use of a small-diameter scanning device with an operative endoscope. There are three types available. Two types of rotating transducers to be used with an operative endoscope for scanning narrower lumen, such as those of the choledochus, pancreatic duct, or stenotic GI tract, caused by advanced carcinoma and cicatrization following inflammations due to various causes. The third type is the manually operated point-probe method of Silverstein and others [17, 22], which was made available by a commercial firm recently. These sonoendoscopes with small transducers, however, invariably suffer from limited penetration and lesser degree of resolution due to the small aperture of the transducer.

The series of equipment developed until now seem to have solved almost all the problems experienced in the past, and the method has established itself

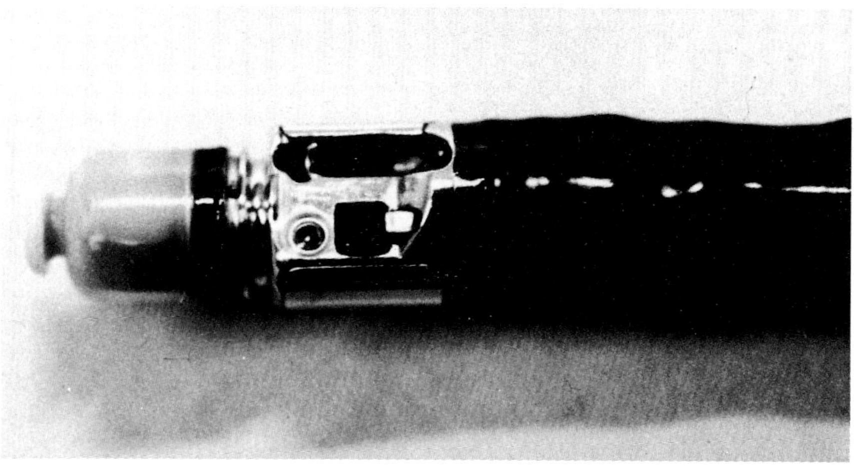

Fig. 3. Scanning head of transduodenal scanner of JFUM3. For the ease of insertion to the duodenal loop, the scanhead is smaller than other scopes and equipped with the biopsy channel for either biopsy or ERCP cannulation

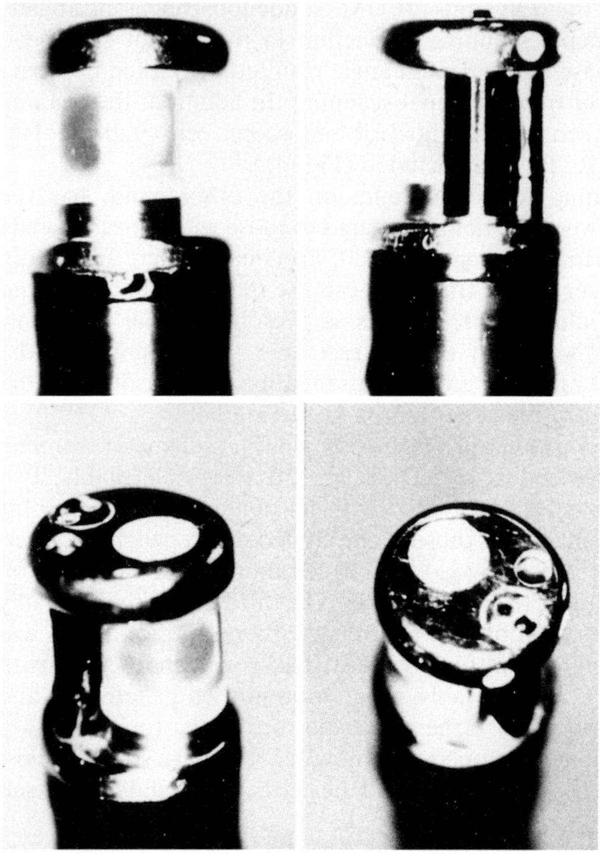

Fig. 4. The scanning head of sonocolonofiberscope. The diameter of the scanhead is larger because of fiberoptics at the very front of the scope. Because of this construction, for the safe insertion of the scope deep to the ascending colon the scan angle of the sonogram is reduced to 300°

as the tool for advanced imaging diagnosis of the GI tract. Thus the application of EUS has diversified and covers practically any area that the sonoendoscope can reach.

Examination Method

As premedication, nervous individuals may require mild sedation, usually injection of antispasmodic agents, prior to examination; combined with an explanation of the examination, this should be sufficient. Following premedication and local anesthesia, the EUS examination proceeds in the following steps:

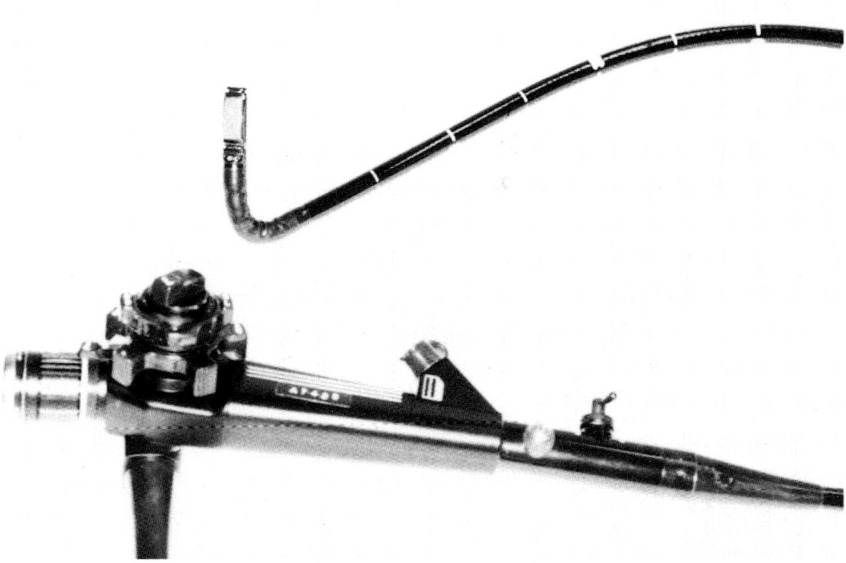

Fig. 5. The convex array type of sonoendoscope, prototype equipment. This scope provides either electronic sector B-mode image or two-dimensional color flow Doppler image when used with the conventional ultrasonic scanner of Aloka SSD 680 scanner

Stomach

1. Insertion of the scope in left decubital position
2. Change of positioning to right decubital position
3. Fill-up of gastric lumen with degassed water
4. Sequential recording of 360° radial scan image
5. Change of positioning to left decubital position
6. Additional infusion of degassed water
7. Sequential recording from angulus to esophagus

Examination steps (Esophagus, duodenum and Colon)

Esophagus

1. Insertion in left decubital position
2. Proceed to cardiac portion and inflate rubber balloon with water
3. Start scanning and record 360° radial scan images

Duodenum

1. Insertion in left decubital position
2. Proceed to pyrolus and pass the ring to duodenum
3. Reaching duodenal papilla, inflate rubber balloon with water
4. Start scanning in duodenal lumen to pylorus

Colon

1. Insertion in left decubital position
2. Start scanning after filling intestinal lumen with water or inflating balloon with water

The EUS images should be recorded in videotape.

Indications

The diagnostic indications for EUS are expanding rapidly. Its established uses are in the following:

Stomach
- Staging of gastric cancer
- Submucosal tumors
- Gastric ulcer, benign and malignant
- Gastric varices
- Assessment of therapeutic result of carcinostatic agent

Esophagus and mediastinum
- Staging of esophageal cancer
- Esophageal tumors
- Mediastinal tumors
- Scanning of heart
- Assessment of aortic wall
- Esophageal varices

Pancreas and biliary tree
- Pancreatitis and pancreas stone
- Staging of pancreatic cancer
- Cystic pancreatic masses
- Obstructive jaundice
- Peripancreatic lymph nodes
- Assessment of duodenal papilla
- Submucosal tumors
- Bile duct cancer

Liver (laparoscopic ultrasound)
- Liver masses, differentiation
- Gallbladder tumors
- Porta hepatis
- Intraperitoneal tumors, localization and characterization

Pathologic Findings

The sonographic appearance of the normal GI is almost identical over the entire length, the tubular structure of the wall consisting of the mucosa, submucosa, muscularis propria with the serosal layers, and the outermost layer (Fig. 6). It is now well established that the stomach wall shows five distinct layers by endosonography. A number of published reports have confirmed that the innermost layer, with increased echogenicity and a thin

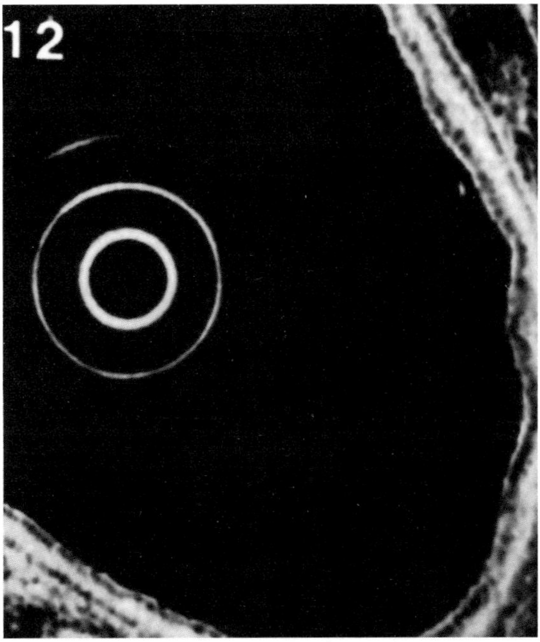

Fig. 6. The normal gastric wall scanned by 12-MHz transducer in the water-filled up stomach. From the innermost, the mucosa, submucosa (echogenic band), hypoechoic muscularis propria, and the thin echogenic serosal layer are visualized. *Circle at left,* the position of the scanhead

hypoechoic layer immediately beneath it, corresponds mainly to the mucosa and partly to the muscularis mucosae, and that the next echogenic layer corresponds to the submucosa. The fourth, hypoechoic layer is the muscularis propria layer, and the outermost, echogenic layer is the serosal layer [1, 3, 18, 19, 30].

Gastric Diseases

Extragastric Compression. Elucidation of the exact cause of extragastric compression is often difficult with routine gastrofiberscopy. EUS examination can readily demonstrate most of the underlying causes of compression. Examples include enlargement of the left lobe of the liver, polycystic kidneys, enlarged spleen or splenic masses, and pancreatic tumors. EUS can solve diagnostic problems more simply than routine abdominal sonography because of the direct imaging and the increased resolution given by high-frequency transducers.

Gastric Submucosal Tumors. Leiomyoma is the most common of submucosal tumors, and its location in relation to layers of the normal gastric mucosa can be identified with EUS. These tumors sometimes reach considerable size without causing specific subjective symptoms. Sonographically, the diagnosis of gastric submucosal tumor is made by demonstrating the echogenic submucosal layer over the tumor and a thin hypoechoic layer or a slit separating it from extragastric organs (Fig. 7) [2, 30, 35]. Typically the masses are round or elliptical in shape and have low-level internal echoes. These may show a marked degree of inhomogeneity in internal texture, generally caused by the central liquefaction that is characteristic of leimyoma. By contrast, an extragastric mass always demonstrates the full thickness of the gastric wall structures over the mass. Respiratory movement of the tumor during real-time imaging often allows better localization of the origin of the tumor.

Malignant Tumors of the Stomach. Among malignant tumors of the stomach, the most frequently encountered is gastric carcinoma. In advanced carcino-

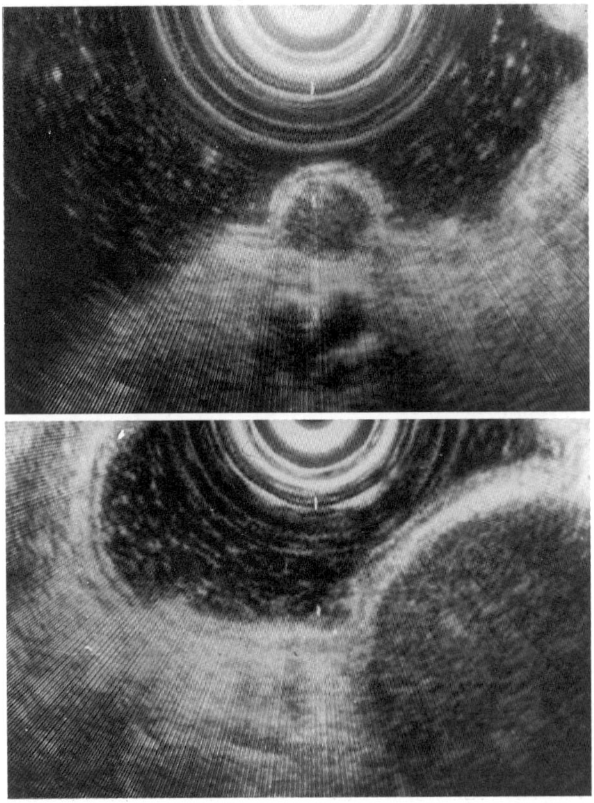

Fig. 7. Cross-sectional images of benign leimyomas. The smaller and larger tumors exhibit entirely identical appearance, a hypoechoic central tumor encircled by the echogenic submucosa. The tumor mass shows connection to the muscularis propria layer, which appears as the thin hypoechoic layer outside of the echogenic submucosal layer

ma, the pseudokidney sign may be manifest even in routine ultrasound. Much smaller masses, however, can only be identified by sonoendoscopy (Fig. 8). Carcinoma in a less advanced stage is generally identified as localized thickening of the gastric wall with distortion or complete destruction of gastric mucosal layer structures. Not infrequently an echogenic ulcer crater is found at the center of the echo-poor carcinoma. Metastatic lymph nodes may be visualized in the vicinity of the mass, as shown in Fig. 9.

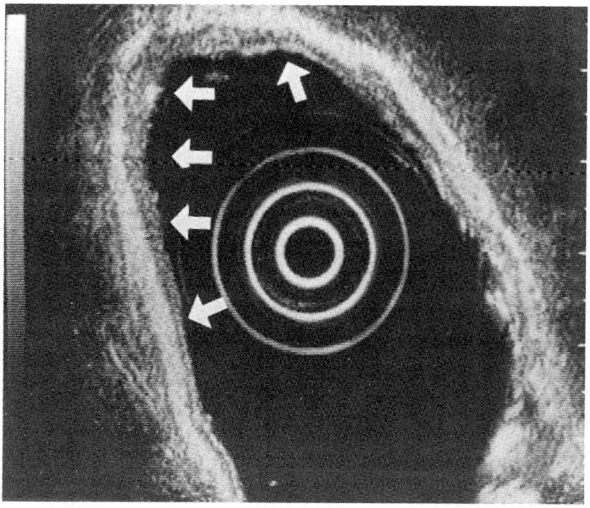

Fig. 8. Ultrasonotomogram of gastric cancer of submucosa type. *Arrows,* supperficially spreading early gastric cancer infiltrating into the submucosal layer, which is an echogenic layer encircling the tumor mass

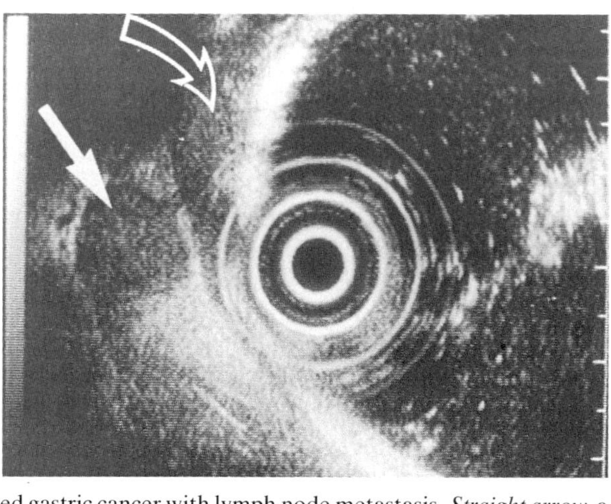

Fig. 9. Tomogram of advanced gastric cancer with lymph node metastasis. *Straight arrow,* a rounded, hypoechoic metastatic lymph node; *curved arrow,* primary gastric cancer, which appears as hypoechoic mass

Table 2. Diagnostic accuracy of EUS for discriminating early versus advanced gastric cancer

EUS diagnosis	Histological diagnosis				Total
	M	SM	PM	SS	
M	**14**	**5**			19
SM	**10**	**23**			33
PM	5	9	**14**	**6**	34
SS			**3**	**22**	25
Total		66		45	111
Accuracy rate		78.8 %		100 %	87.4 %

M, Mucosal cancer; SM, cancer remains at the depth of submucosa; PM, advanced cancer infiltrating to propria muscle layer; SS, advanced cancer beyond subserosal layer

Due to the marked improvement in spatial as well as contrast resolution of sonoendoscopy, it is now possible to apply the technique to the staging of gastric carcinoma. The T1 carcinoma, that of the mucosal type or that extending to the submucosal layer is clearly differentiated from those of more advanced (T2,T3) stages. There is a high correlation between sonoendoscopic and histopathologic diagnosis, as shown in Table 2. If a lesion is not complicated with ulceration, nearly 100 % accuracy in discriminating early versus advanced gastric carcinoma can be achieved. A comparative study at our institution also revealed that the diagnostic accuracy of cancer staging depends largely on the resolution of the equipment used. Discriminating accuracy between early versus advanced carcinoma was definitely higher in the series examined by the dual transducer system GFUM3/EUM3 equipped with 7.5- and 12-MHz disc transducers compared to the series examined by the single transducer system of 10 MHz (Table 3) [24].

A less frequent type of malignant gastric tumor, lymphoma, is seen as a discrete hypoechoic tumor mass or as diffuse thickening of the gastric wall. Lymphomatous mass lesion may be accompanied by a slight degree of erosion or even deep ulceration, depending upon the grades of mucosal involvement [2, 11, 12, 31]. Direct visualization of the cross-sectional image of the lymphomatous infiltration not infrequently serves as an accurate indicator of the therapeutic effects of anticancer chemotherapy.

Identification of Gastric Varices. The occurrence of gastric varices may be found either with or without concomitant esophageal varices. Endoscopically, mucosal varices are easily identified by their characteristic endoscopic findings, especially if they are very apparent. In questionable cases, EUS is strongly recommended because of the ease of identification: the presence of anechoic chains of engorged vessels with blood flow connecting to the deeper vessels also engorged as collaterals.

Table 3. Diagnostic accuracy of EUS for discriminating early versus advanced gastric cancer

EUS diagnosis	Histological diagnosis				Total
	M	SM	PM	SS	
GFUM2/EUM2					
M	**8**	**4**			12
SM	**3**	**9**			12
PM	4	8	**12**	**4**	28
SS			**1**	**16**	17
Total	36		33		69
Accuracy rate	66.7 %		100 %		82.6 %
GFUM3/EUM3					
M	**6**	**1**			7
SM	**7**	**14**			21
PM	1	1	**2**	**2**	6
SS			**2**	**6**	8
Total	30		12		42
Accuracy rate	93.3 %		100 %		95.2 %

M, Mucosal cancer; SM, cancer remains at the depth of submucosa; PM, advanced cancer infiltrating to propria muscle layer; SS, advanced cancer beyond subserosal layer

Diseases of the Esophagus

EUS of the esophagus is technically much simpler than that in other parts of the GI tract. The use of the balloon method is often necessary becaue of the limited size of the esophageal lumen.

The diagnostic applications of esophageal EUS are similar to those in the stomach, the major ones being differential diagnosis of tumors and staging of esophagenal malignancies. Mucosal cancer confined to the very surface of the mucosa is often difficult to image because of the nearfield phenomenon. However, interpretation of carcinomatous infiltration is precise, including assessment of invasion to the thoracic aorta or the involvement of regional lymph nodes. The findings are frequently very helpful in interpreting resectability of the mass preoperatively.

Benign lesions, leiomyomas, and cysts are readily identified by their characteristic sonographic findings. Diagnosis of esophageal varices has been well documented [5].

Diseases of the Pancreas and Biliary System

The pancreas and biliary tree can be imaged by transgastric or transduodenal scanning [9, 36, 37]. The former method is similar to the maneuver described in the previous section on gastric scanning, and the gallbladder and pancreas

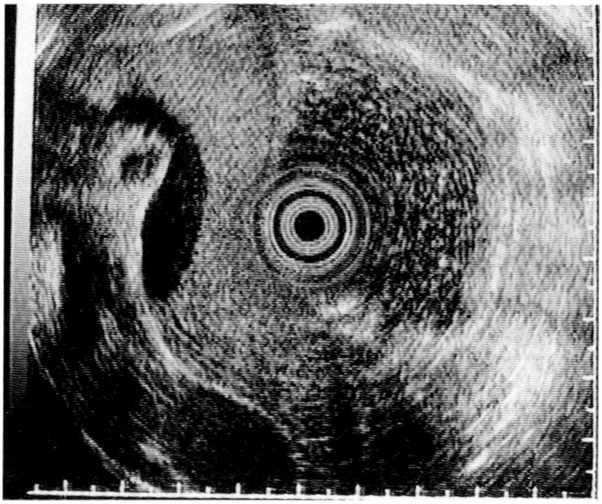

Fig. 10. The normal pancreas scanned by transgastric scanning. A part of the pancreatic head, full image of the body, and a part of the tail are imaged *(left)*. Splenic vein, superior mesenteric artery, and a part of the left kidney are also imaged

can be imaged by placing the scan head in the pylorus or antrum of the stomach, respectively. The shape, location, and characteristic internal texture identify the organ (Fig. 10). Detailed cross-sectional images of the lower part of the common duct and the head of the pancreas can be obtained by inserting the tip of the scope into the descending duodenum having the inflated balloon covering the scanning compartment [36, 37].

Among the indications (see above), the identification of malignant tumors is of prime importance by virtue of the resolving power of the method in defining the location and size of the tumor mass lesion and the presence or absence of invasion or dissemination. The method is particularly suited for early detection of pancreatic carcinoma, including that arising in the tail, and carcinoma of the gallbladder or bile duct at sites that are difficult to image [6, 14, 29, 36, 37]. Benign tumors can also be diagnosed with considerable accuracy. Cysts and stones are instantly diagnosed on the basis of their sonographic characteristics. The diagnosis of pancreatic carcinoma at the tail and tumors obstructing the main pancreatic duct is simple and accurate compared to routine transabdominal ultrasound (Figs. 11, 12).

Intraduodenal scanning is more effective in defining the lower portion of the common duct and the papilla of Vater, where it has proven superior to imaging by the transgastric route.

Tumor-forming chronic pancreatitis frequently poses difficult diagnostic problems especially in regard to differentiation from pancreatic carcinoma; however, EUS is frequently able to differentiate changes characteristic to pancreatic carcinoma based on the lack of a specific echo pattern.

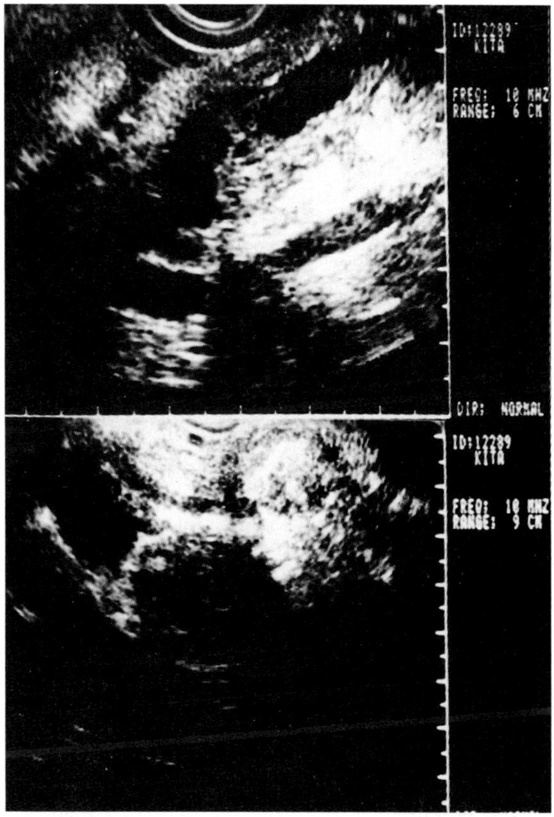

Fig. 11. Carcinoma of the pancreas, head. *Above*, enlarged main pancreatic duct; *below*, hypoechoic tumor at the head of the pancreas

Diseases of the Colon

Routine sonographic examination of the rectum and sigmoid colon requires meticulous techniques, including water enema and body positioning, to yield satisfactory diagnostic imaging. The purpose of sonography here is similar to that in the upper GI tract, namely for clinical staging of colonic malignancies, since it demonstrates the size, extent of tumor infiltration, and even dissemination to adjacent organs or lymph nodes [3, 18, 26] (Fig. 13). It can also be used for the differentiation between benign and malignant tumors, intramural and extramural changes, involvement of the colon by nonmalignant diseases such as periproctal abscesses, bleeding, Crohn's disease, and tumor invasion from outside of the colon.

Endosonography can be used effectively for scanning of the entire parts of the colon and rectum either alone or combined with endoscopy. The balloon method ensures complete contact of the scanhead to the wall of the large

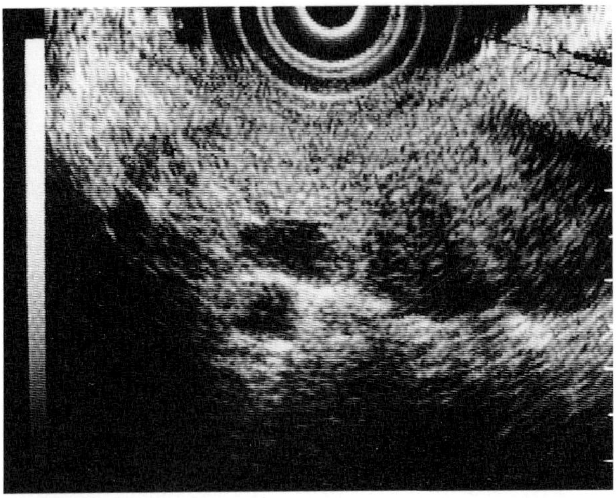

Fig. 12. Carcinoma of the pancreas, tail. A hypoechoic tumor mass at the tail of the pancreas is demonstrated as ill-marginated mass (right). The size of the mass in this cross-section is 1.6 × 4 cm

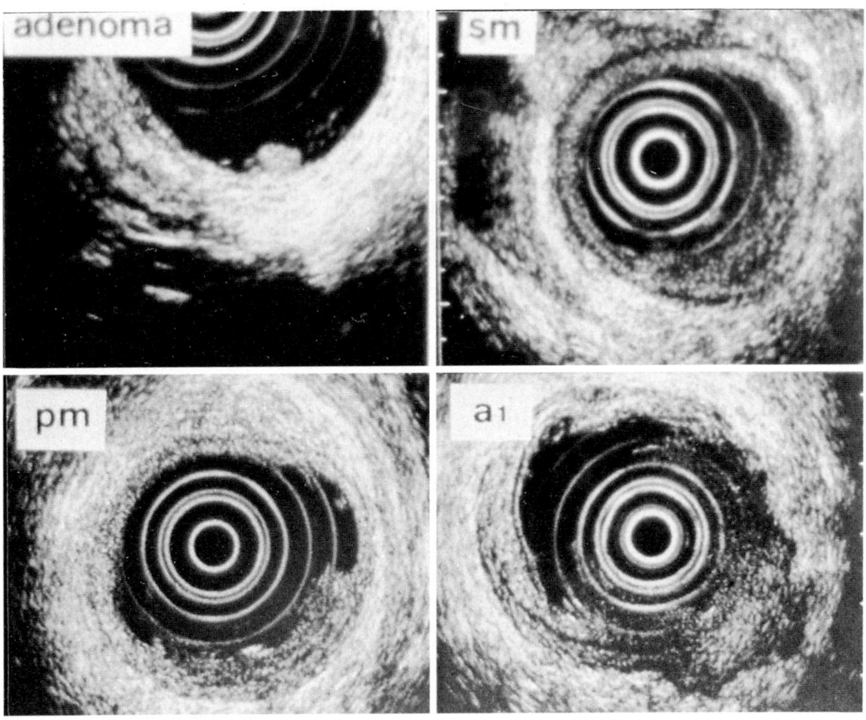

Fig. 13. Tomograms of colonic cancer with different stages. *Upper left,* adenoma, benign; *upper right,* early-stage submucosal cancer; *lower left,* advanced cancer, invading the muscularis propria layer; *lower right,* advanced cancer of a1 stage

intestine in the same way as in the esophagus. Either mechanical or electronic scanning systems may be used for examination of the rectum; however, for the other part of the colon, use of the sonocolonofiberscope is mandatory to avoid any accident due to blind insertion of the equipment. Sonograms of the normal rectum wall and those of the colon also have the five-layer structure common to the other parts of the GI tract.

The Scanning Technique. After pretreatment of the patient, similarly as in colonoscopy, the tip of the scope covered by the rubber balloon is inserted into the rectal lumen. Using a technique similar to that in routine colonoscopy, the tip of the scope is advanced with continuous inflation of the lumen by air and under the inspection through fiberoptics prepared at the frontal plane of the scope. When the scope reaches the cecum, the balloon covering the tip of the scope is inflated by water, and ultrasonic scanning is started. The EUS images are recorded on videotape continuously during examination.

In the EUS examination of the colon and rectum, the diagnostic capability and image quality produced are definitely superior in the mechanical scanner for the same reasons as in EUS examination of the upper GI tract.

Formerly, the indication for EUS was limited to diseases of the rectum; however, the introduction of ultrasono-colonofiberscopes has extended the area of examination to the entire length of the colon.

Our preliminary study as well as reports by others have amply demonstrated that the staging of colonic carcinoma is so accurate that EUS can be justified as one of the standard techniques in assessing wall invasion by colonic carcinoma (T factors). For the N factor – evaluation of lymph node metastasis – there are certain limitations inherent to the instrument used and to scanning techniques.

Laparoscopic Ultrasonography for the Examination of Liver Diseases

Sonographic examination of localized lesions of the liver has advanced rapidly following the widespread use of high-resolution real-time ultrasound. The method has resulted in the detection of early-stage liver cancer and cases with small liver masses of indeterminate pathology. To resolve these difficult differential diagnostic problems, a special method using laparoscopic ultrasound has been introduced [10, 13].

Two different kinds of sonolaparoscopes are available, one with mechanical and the other with a linear-array electronic scanner (Figs. 14, 15). The former employs a rotating mirror to avoid the nearfield phenomenon and to obtain good resolution in areas close to the scanning head. Either instrument employs an optical unit to observe the tip of the scope during the insertion into the abdominal cavity via a trocar to avoid trauma to the intraperitoneal organs. The scanning compartment is placed gently onto the surface of the

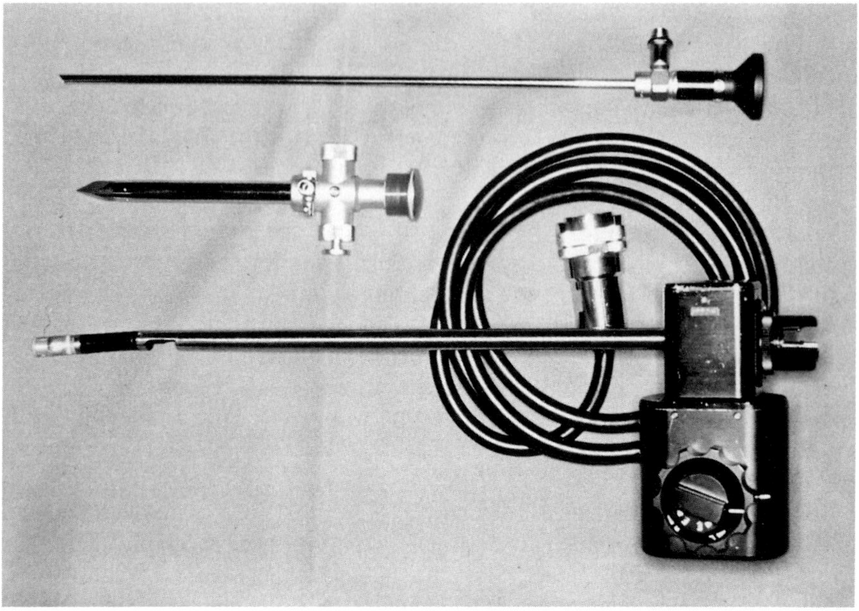

Fig. 14. The radial scanning sonolaparoscope with trocar. This scope provides 180° radial scan images with the 10-MHz disc transducer fixed at the scanhead. Scanning is performed by a rotating ultrasonic mirror in the scanhead

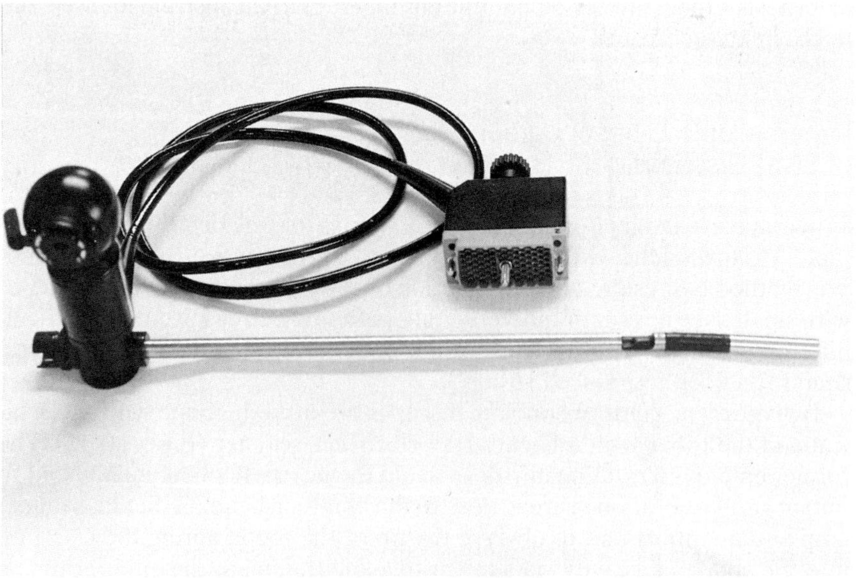

Fig. 15. The linear-scanning sonolaparoscope, prototype

liver and moved across its surface to locate the lesion. If a doubtful lesion is identified, sonographic images are recorded on videotape.

The high-resolution images yielded by high-frequency transducers are particularly powerful means for accurate diagnosis of mass lesions in the liver.

As is shown in Figs. 16, 17, hepatocellular carcinoma is clearly differentiated from cavernous hemangioma based on its characteristic sonographic findings. The information supplied by this technique is not limited to the cross-sectional images of the tumor but extends to the feeding vessels of the tumor, which is valuable in planning surgery.

The high-resolution image of liver tumors not only provides information in regards to its location; qualitative differential diagnosis can also be made based upon ultrasonic texture changes, shape and posterior echo enhancement, and compression signs to the periphery. All of these are frequently very powerful means of differential diagnosis. In selected cases, however, biopsy of liver tissue guided by sonolaparoscopy have been reported as successful in differentiating malignant tumors from benign conditions such as hyperplastic nodule, focal nodular hyperplasia, hemangioma, and adenomatous hyperplasias.

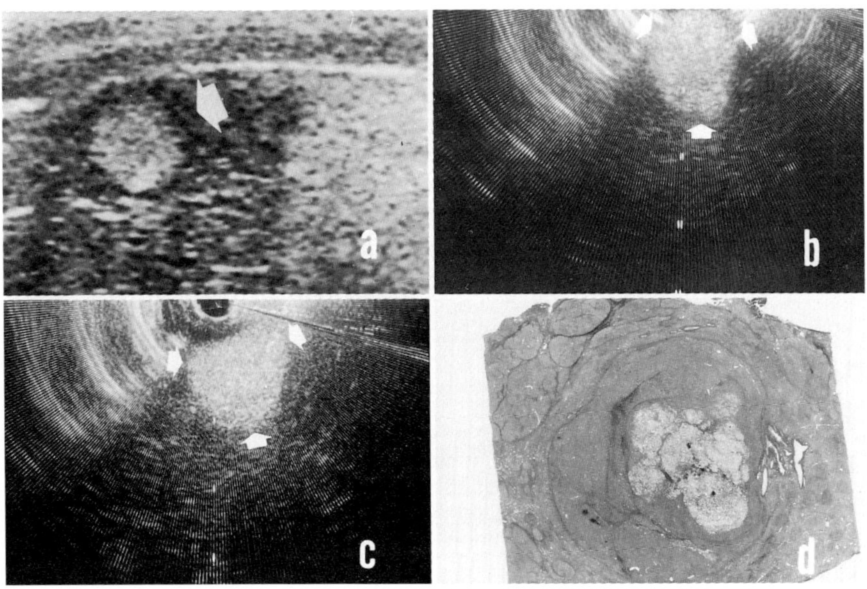

Fig. 16a – d. Sonogram of hepatocellular carcinoma by sonolaparoscope of radial scanning type. **a** Echogenic tumor detected by routine ultrasound. **b, c** Sonolaparoscopic images with irregularly outlined tumor of highly echogenic nature. **d** Extirpated tumor mass with central fatty changes (H&E stain). *Arrows,* tumor mass

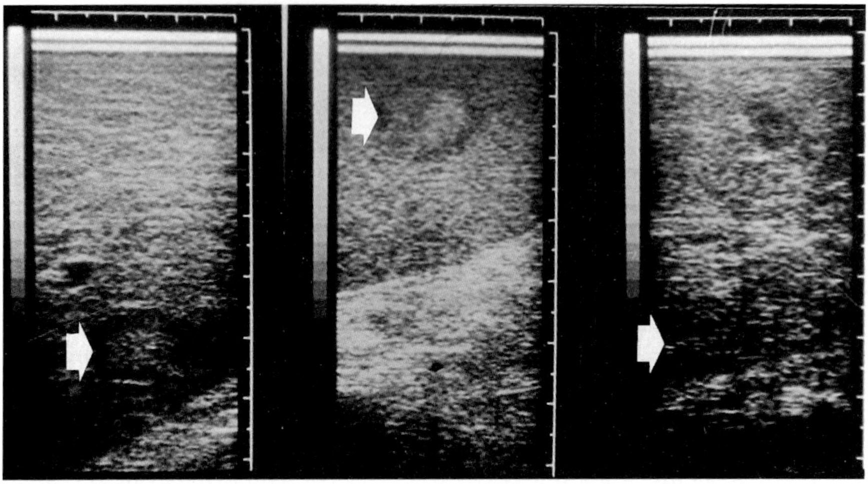

Fig. 17. Small hepatocellular carcinoma demonstrated by the linear scanning type of sonolaparoscope. *Arrows*, small liver cancer with typical sonographic appearance

Conclusion

The method of endoscopic sonography is still a relatively new technique. However, the speed of development of equipment and fundamental technology is so unexpectedly swift that soon EUS will show significant expansion in its diagnostic application, both for the upper and the lower GI tract and for pancreato-biliary diseases.

The method is safe and reasonably tolerable to the patient. High resolution of EUS imaging gives clear-cut and accurate diagnostic information on the GI tract which cannot be obtained by routine ultrasonography.

Additional use of biopsy and two-dimensional color flow Doppler methods from within the lumen of the GI tract will bring the most potent diagnostic capability to the method.

References

1. Aibe T, Fujii T, Okita K et al. (1986) A fundamental study of normal layer structure of the gastrointestinal wall visualized by endoscopic ultrasonography. Scand J Gastroenterol Suppl 123: 6–15
2. Aibe T, Takemoto T (1988) Benign lesions of the gastrointestinal tract, intestinal tract. In: Kawai K (ed) Endoscopic ultrasound in gastroenterology. Igakushoin, Tokyo, pp 44–55
3. Bolondi L, Caletti G, Casanova P et al. (1986) Problems and variations in the interpretation of the ultrasound feature of the normal upper and lower GI tract wall. Scand J Gastroenterol Suppl 123: 16–26
4. Caletti G, Bolondi L, Labo G (1984) Ultrasonic endoscopy. The gastrointestinal wall. Scand J Gastroenterol Suppl 102: 5–8

5. Caletti G, Bolondi L, Zani L et al. (1986) Detection of portal hypertension and esophageal varices by means of endoscopic ultrasonography. Scand J Gastroenterol Suppl 123: 74–77
6. Classen M, Lutz H et al. (1984) Pancreatic pseudocysts and tumors in endosonography. Scand J Gastroenterol Suppl 94: 77–84
7. Dancygier H, Classen M (1986) Sonoendoscopic diagnosis of benign pancreatic and biliary lesions. Scand J Gastroenterol Suppl 123: 119–122
8. Di Magno EP, Buxton JL, Regan PT et al. (1980) Ultrasonic endo-scopy. Lancet 1: 629–631
9. Fukuda M, Nakano Y, Saito K et al. (1984) Endoscopic ultrasonography in diagnosis of pancreatic carcinoma. The use of a liquid-filled stomach method. Scand J Gastroenterol Suppl 94: 65–76
10. Fukuda M, Mima S, Tanabe T, Haniu T, Suzuki Y, Hirata K, Terada S (1984) Endoscopic sonography of the liver – diagnostic application of the echolaparoscope locating intrahepatic lesions. Scand J Gastroenterol Suppl 102: 24–38
11. Fukuda M (1984) Use of the echoendoscopoe and echolaparoscope in the diagnosis of intraabdominal cancer. Intraluminal scanning. In: Kossoff G, Fukuda M (eds) Ultrasonic differential diagnosis of tumors. Igakushoin, New York, pp 186–199
12. Fukuda M (1985) Endoscopic ultrasonography. In: Gill RW, Dadd MJ (eds) Proceedings of the 4th meeting of the World Federation for Ultrasound in Medicine and Biology. Pergamon, Sydney, pp 13–16
13. Fukuda M (1986) Endoscopic sonography: use of the echoendoscope and echolaparoscope in the diagnosis of intra-abdominal disorders. In: Sanders RC, Hill M (eds) Ultrasound annual 1986. Raven, New York, pp 141–170
14. Hayashi Y, Nakazawa S, Kimoto E et al. (1989) Clinicopathologic analysis of endoscopic ultrasonograms in pancreatic mass lesions. Endoscopy 21: 121–125
15. Heyder N, Lux G (1986)Malignant lesions of the upper gastrointestinal tract. Scand J Gastroenterol Suppl 123: 47–51
16. Hisanaga K, Hisanaga A, Hibi N et al. (1980) High speed rotation scanner for transesophageal sectional echocardiography. Am J Cardiol 46: 837–842
17. Ito K, Fukuda M, Hirata K, Mitani M et al. (1989) B-mode image of the normal gastrointestinal tract: analysis of wall structure by high-frequency point probe system. Proc JSUM 55: 491–492
18. Kimmey MB, Silverstein FE, Martin RW (1988) Ultrasound interaction with the intestinal wall: esophagus, stomach and colon. In: Kawai K (ed) Endoscopic ultrasonography in gastroenterology. Igakushoin, Tokyo, pp 35–43
19. Kimmey MB, Haggitt RC (1989) Histologic correlates of gastrointestinal wall. Gastroenterology 96: 433–441
20. Lees WR (1986) Endoscopic ultrasonography of chronic pancreatitis and pancreatic pseudocysts. Scand J Gastroenterol Suppl 123: 123–129
21. Lux G, Heyder N (1986) Endoscopic ultrasonography of the pancreas: technical aspects. Scand J Gastroenterol Suppl 123: 112–118
22. Martin RW, Silverstein FE, Kimmey MB (1989) A 20-MHz ultrasound system for imaging the intestinal wall. Ultrasound Med Biol: 273–280
23. Natori H, Tamaki S, Izumi S, Yoshita Y, Kira S (1983) Clinical application of ultrasonic endoscope using linear array transducer of the diseases of the mediastinum. In: Lerski A, Morley P (eds) Ultrasound '82. Pergamon, Oxford, pp 339–343
24. Mitani M, Hirata K (1990) Studies on staging of gastric cancer by endoscopic ultrasonography. Sapporo Med J 59: 615–627
25. Rifkin MD, Gordon SJ (1986) Sonoendoscopic evaluation of extraesophageal and extragastric abnormalities: review. Scand J Gastroenterol Suppl 123: 68–73
26. Rifkin MD, McGlynn ET, Marks G (1986) Endorectal sonographic retrospective staging of rectal cancer. Scand J Gastroenterol Suppl 123: 99–103
27. Sasai T (1988) Development of ultrasonic endoscope. In: Kawai K (ed) Endoscopic ultrasonography in gastroenterology. Igakushoin, Tokyo, pp. 18–34

28. Tio TL, Tytgat GNJ (1983) Endoscopic ultrasonography in the assessment of intra- and transmural infiltration of tumours in the esophagus stomach, and papilla of Vater and in the detection of extraesophageal lesions. Endoscopy 16: 203–210
29. Tio TL, Tytgat GNJ (1986) Endoscopic ultrasonography of bile duct malignancy and the preoperative assessment of local resectability. Scand J Gastroenterol Suppl 123: 151–157
30. Tio TL, Tytgat GNJ (1986) Endoscopic sonography of normal and pathologic upper gastrointestinal wall structure. Comparison of studies in vivo and in vitro with histology. Scand J Gastroenterol Suppl 123: 27–33
31. Tio TL, Jager DH, Tytgat GNJ (1986) Endoscopic ultrasound in detecton and staging of gastric non-Hodgkin lymphoma. Scand J Gastroenterol Suppl 123: 52–58
32. Tanaka Y, Yasuda K, Aibe T et al. (1984) Anatomical and pathological aspects in ultrasonic endoscopy of GI tract. Scand J Gastroenterol Suppl 94: 43–50
33. Wild JJ, Reid JM (1955) Echographic tissue diagnosis. Proceedings of the 4th annual conference on ultrasonic therapy. Detroit, 27 August 1955
34. Wild JJ, Reid JM (1957) Progress in techniques of soft tissue examination by 15 MC pulsed ultrasound. In: Kelly E (ed) Ultrasound in biology and medicine. American Institute of Biological Sciences, Washington DC, pp 30–45
35. Yasuda K, Nakajima M, Kawai K (1986) Endoscopic ultrasonography in the diagnosis of submucosal tumor of the upper GI tract. Scand J Gastroenterol Suppl 123: 59–67
36. Yasuda K, Nakajima M, Mukai H et al. (1987) The detection of small pancreatic cancers by endoscopic ultrasonography (EUS). In: Dancygier H, Classen M (eds) 5th international symposium on endoscopic ultrasonography. Demeter, Graefelfing, pp 86–91
37. Yasuda K, Nakajima M, Kawai K (1988) Malignant lesions of the gastro intestinal tract. In: Kawai K (ed) Endoscopic ultrasound in gastroenterology. Igakushoin, Tokyo, pp 56–71

Doppler Flowmetry in Portal Hypertension

L. Bolondi, S. Gaiani, and L. Barbara

Clinical applications of Doppler flowmetry of hepatic vessels include assessment of the presence, direction, and characteristics of blood flow. Quantitative measurement of the volume of blood flow has also been attempted in some of the major abdominal arteries and veins, and this possibility is awakening increasing interest; however the reliability of these measurements is still questioned. Otherwise, the qualitative information about flow pattern provided by the Doppler investigation is no longer in question, since it not only contributes to clarifying doubtful images in real-time ultrasonography but also provides new insights in many clinical conditions.

Detection of Blood Flow

The presence of blood flow moving within the portal vein is the simplest Doppler finding to ascertain. The diagnosis of portal vein obstruction is sometimes uncertain in real-time ultrasound imaging, especially in cases of

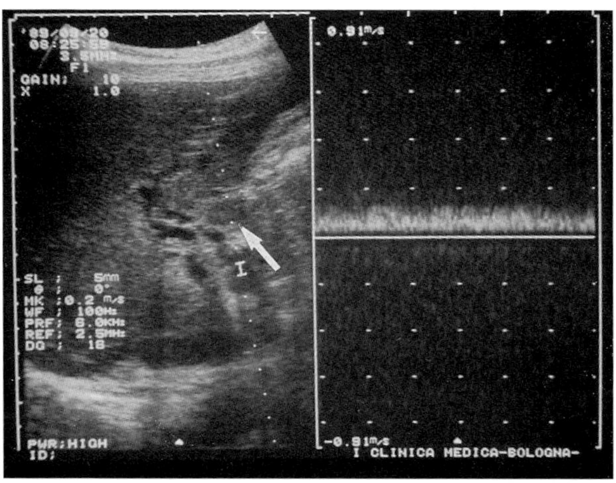

Fig. 1. Partial thrombosis of the portal vein. The flat Doppler signal above the reference line indicates the presence of a venous flow toward the liver *(arrow)*. *Right,* intercostal scan

recent thrombosis, when the echo pattern of the thrombus is markedly hypoechoic and may be missed, so that the lumen appears to be patent. In these cases the absence of the Doppler signal from the portal vein confirms the diagnosis. In other instances the finding of the Doppler signal can contribute to distinguishing a partial thrombosis (Fig. 1) from a complete obstruction, where no signal can be detected at the porta hepatis. For this purpose Doppler flowmetry may be even more accurate than arterioportography, which can erroneously suggest portal thrombosis in the case of complete diversion of the contrast medium into large portosystemic collaterals [7]. Liver cirrhosis is the most important cause of thrombosis of the portal vein. The incidence of this complication is unclear, since an old autoptic series [19] reports a 11 % whereas a more recent angiographic study shows an

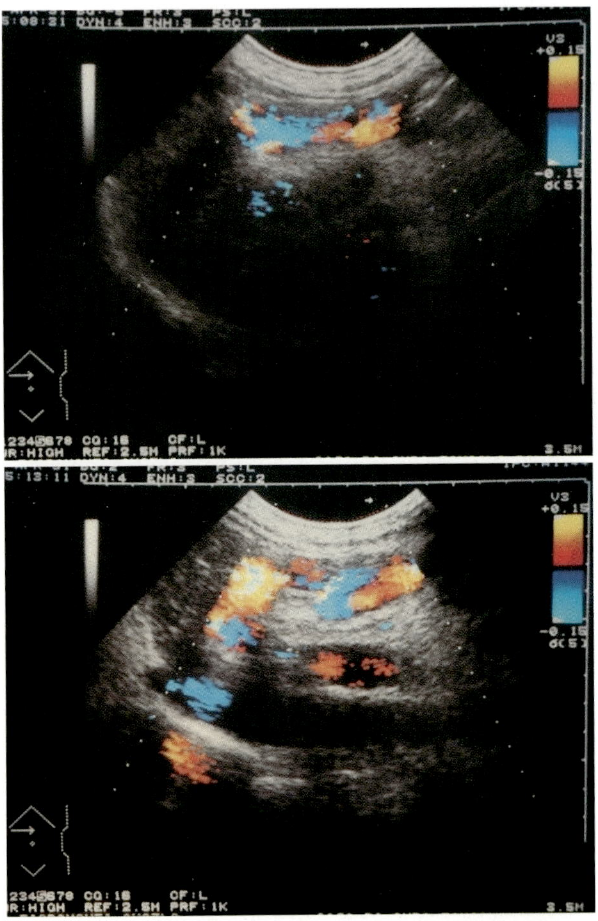

Fig. 2. Patent and dilated paraumbilical vein showing a turbulent flow upon color Doppler. *Above,* the vessel runs in the deep abdominal layers; *below,* origin of the paraumbilical vein from a dilated left portal branch. Longitudinal scans at the epigastrium

incidence of about 1 % [28]. The extensive application of Doppler ultrasound flowmetry in nonselected patients affected by liver cirrhosis contributed to clarifying the prevalence of partial and complete portal thrombosis, which has recently been estimated to be 5.7 % and 1.8 %, respectively [15].

Pulsed Doppler and color flow mapping may also be helpful in identifying flow in collateral vessels which often develop as a consequence of portal hypertension (Figs. 2–4, 5b).

Direction of Blood Flow

This is another unequivocal qualitative finding provided by Doppler ultrasound. Its importance in the investigation of hepatic hemodynamics is striking. There are conflicting data regarding the prevalence of a reversed flow in the portal venous system in liver cirrhosis. Previous studies, using angiographic techniques, report a rate of reversed flow ranging from 0 % to 3.1 % [12, 29, 31] whereas other authors report higher figures (14.8 %) [6]. Therefore, this hemodynamic abnormality is not so uncommon. However, the arteriographic rate of reversed flow may not exactly reflect the prevalence of this abnormality in a nonselected population of cirrhosis patients because only those with complicated portal hypertension and/or candidates for surgery undergo this invasive procedure.

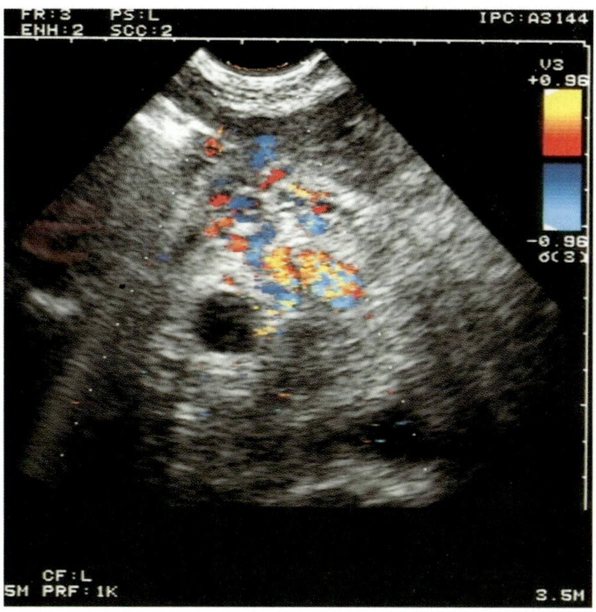

Fig. 3. Thin collateral vessels in the retroperitoneal and pancreatic region. Transverse scan at the epigastrium

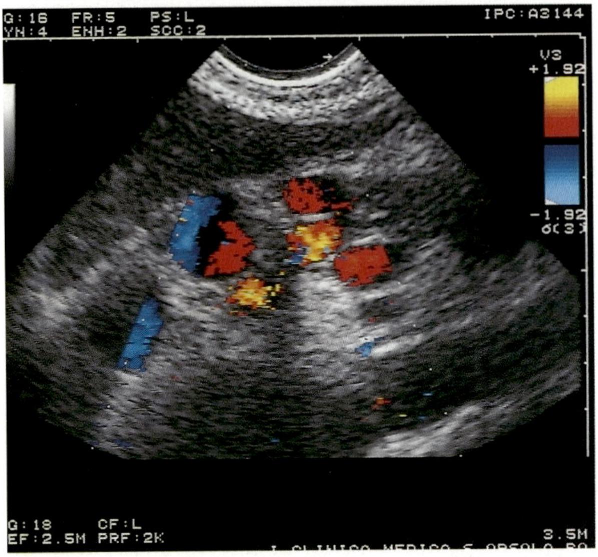

Fig. 4. Large collateral vessels in the gastroesophageal region (posterior to the left liver lobe). Longitudinal scan at the epigastrium

We assessed [15] the direction of blood flow in the portal venous system in 228 consecutive patients affected by histologically confirmed liver cirrhosis. The overall prevalence of hepatofugal flow was 8.3 % (19/228). Hepatofugal flow was detected in seven patients (3.1 %) in the portal trunk, seven (3.1 %) in the splenic vein (Fig. 5a), and in five (2.1 %) in the superior mesenteric vein. Reversal of flow in these vessels is often related to the presence of large portosystemic collaterals such as splenorenal shunts (Fig. 5b). To assess the implication of hepatofugal flow on the risk of bleeding and survival, we prospectively evaluated two groups of patients with hepatofugal and hepatopetal flow in the portal venous system [15]. This study showed a significantly higher rate of bleeding in patients with hepatopetal flow (Fig. 6), thus suggesting a protective role of reversed flow against the risk of variceal bleeding.

Characteristics of Blood Flow and Its Disturbances

One of the most exciting prerogatives of the Doppler signals is that the characteristics of waveform and spectral distribution of frequencies are generally consequences of the hemodynamic factors and location of the vessel. Therefore the pattern of the Doppler signal (and its acoustic characteristics) often allows one to identify its origin, also in circumstances in which the image may be equivocal. It can be said that any vessel has its own "signature", from which it can be recognized [34]. The assessment of flow

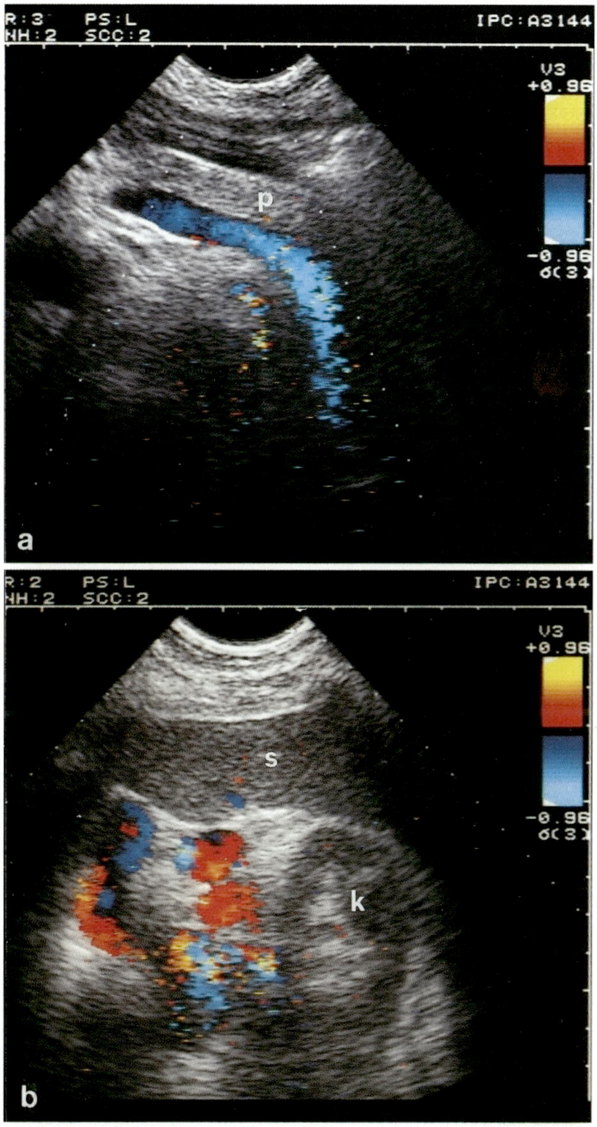

Fig. 5 a, b. Color Doppler of a patient with liver cirrhosis and spontaneous portosystemic shunt. **a** Transverse scan at the epigastrium. **b** Left subcostal scan. In the splenic vein **(a)** the flow is hepatofugal *(blue; arrow)* and is drained by large splenorenal collaterals **(b).** *p*, Pancreas; *s*, spleen; *k*, kidney

disturbances from waveform data includes some semiquantitative methods based on the analysis of the velocity profile and the calculation of the interrelationship between maximum, minimum, and mean frequencies of the spectrum. Numerous indices (pulsatility index, resistance index) have been proposed to describe waveforms of arterial flow. Because it is not necessary to

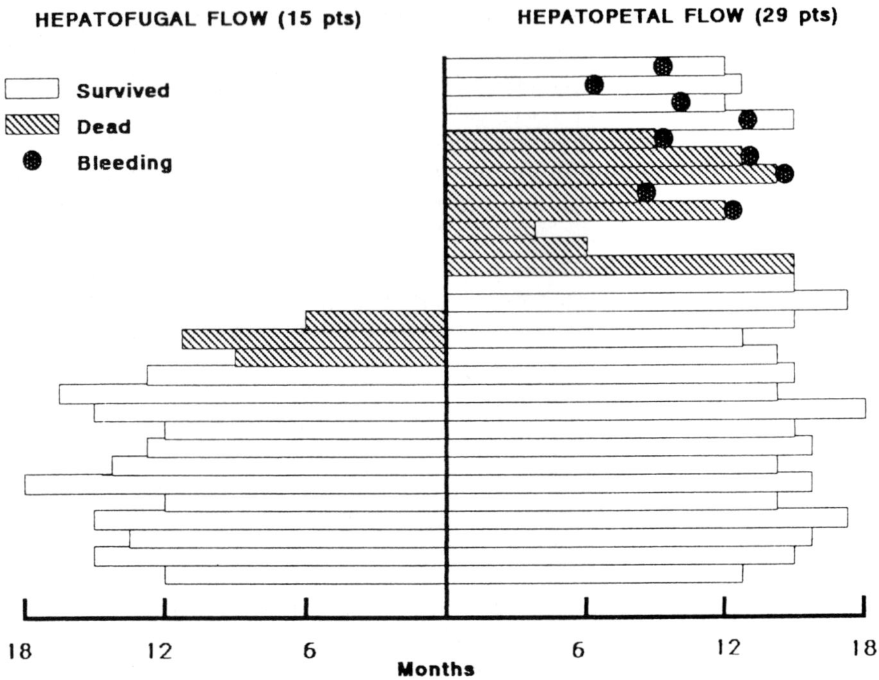

Fig. 6. Clinical outcome in individual cirrhosis patients with hepatopetal and hepatofugal flow detected by Doppler ultrasound in the portal venous system. The survival rate did not significantly differ between the two groups, whereas the occurrence of bleeding was significantly higher in patients with hepatopetal flow (9/29 versus 0/15; $p < 0.02$). (From [15] with permission)

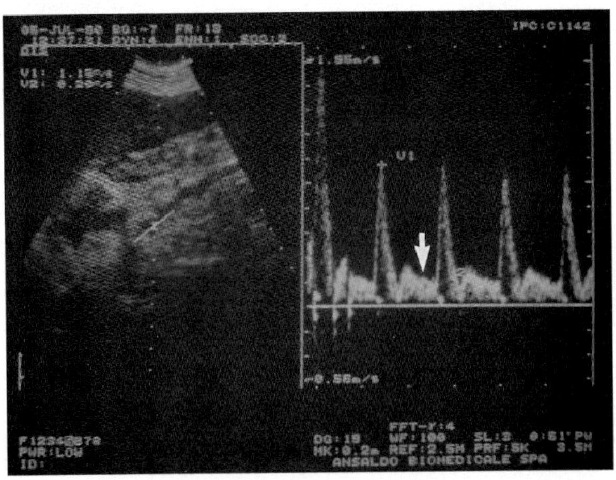

Fig. 7. Superior mesenteric artery in patient with liver cirrhosis shows an increased diastolic flow *(arrow)*. Longitudinal scan at the epigastrium

know the angle of incidence of the ultrasonic beam when calculating one of these indices, they can be assessed in vessels that are too small or tortuous to be imaged (e.g., the intrahepatic arteries). Since pulsatility of an arterial waveform is influenced by the impedance of the distal vascular bed, the investigation of this parameter could be useful in liver diseases.

One of the most striking characteristics of the systemic hemodynamics of cirrhotic patients is the hyperdynamic circulation associated with a fall in arterial resistance. This phenomenon has been studied utilizing the Doppler method by a French group [10] who found that the pulsatility index of the superior mesenteric artery is significantly decreased in patients affected by liver cirrhosis (Fig. 7) and acute hepatitis, but not in cases of portal vein thrombosis unrelated to liver cirrhosis.

Hepatic and splenic arteries normally have a well-represented diastolic component due to a low-resistance peripheral bed. In some episodes of acute rejection of liver transplantation it was noted that the normal diastolic component of the hepatic arterial signal was lost, giving a high-impedance signal [35]. The value of this finding, however, has been subjected to some doubt by further observation [22].

Analysis of the Doppler signals arising from venous structures may also provide interesting data. The hepatic veins in healthy humans display a triphasic waveform depending upon cardiac cycles and particularly the fluctuating right atrial pressure. We have observed that these phasic variations of flow are completely lost (Fig. 8) in 18.3% of cases of liver cirrhosis with portal hypertension and greatly reduced in another 31.7% [3]. The pathophysiology of this behavior is unclear. We have found a significant correlation ($p < 0.01$) with the decrease in the resistance index in the superior mesenteric artery and the increase in the Child-Pugh score. These data suggest that the

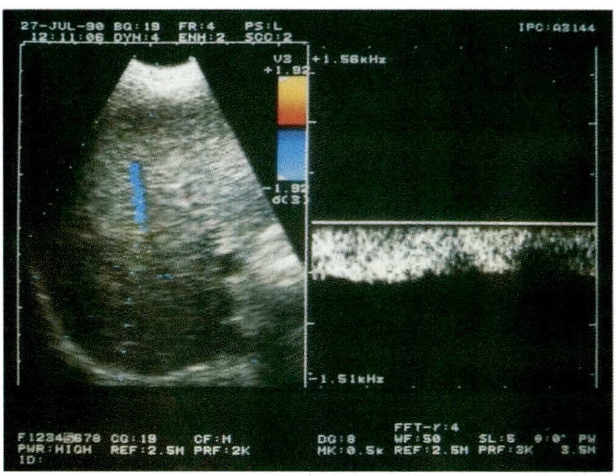

Fig. 8. Flattening of the flow profile in the hepatic vein of a patients with liver cirrhosis. Right intercostal scan

hyperdynamic circulation and the severity of liver tissue alterations could play a role in determining changes in the hepatic vein waveform. Absence, reversal, or steady flow in the hepatic veins may be consistent with the diagnosis of Budd-Chiari syndrome. We have recently demonstrated that these signs, associated with flat or reversed flow in the inferior vena cava, were detectable in 7/8 patients studied [4].

Quantitative Measurement of Blood Flow

Measurement of flow volume has always proved much more difficult. Electromagnetic flowmetry [23, 30], indocyanin green clearance [9], indicator dilution [18], and thermodilution techniques [5] do not completely satisfy the clinical needs. Noninvasive measurements using Doppler ultrasound have therefore attracted a great deal of attention in recent years. This measurement is based on the principle of the uniform insonation method, by which the entire volume of blood in a cross-section of the vessel is exposed to a uniform ultrasonic beam. The instantaneous mean velocity (V) calculated from the mean Doppler shift is multiplied by the cross-sectional area (A) of the vessel, thus giving the volume flow (Q): $Q = VA$.

Possible sources of errors in the quantitative estimates of blood flow in the portal vein have been outlined by Gill [16] and reconsidered by Burns [8], and Dauzat and Pomier [11]. A critical point is the calculation of mean velocity. Its determination from the maximal velocity by a fixed coefficient may be inaccurate because the velocity profile in the portal vein differs from patient to patient. It is therefore necessary to calculate mean velocity directly on the Doppler spectrum, and this can be achieved by the software of recent instrumentation. Regarding the portal vein, its 3- to 4-cm straight course, its quite large caliber, and its oblique position with respect to the abdominal wall are favorable factors for the Doppler investigation. Measurements of mean velocity are to be made on Doppler traces of 4–6 s to avoid eventual flow fluctuations, which are also reduced by examining the patients during suspended respiration.

In a recent paper [32] the intra- and interobserver variability of Doppler ultrasound measurements was assessed in normal volunteers. Intraobserver variability proved low in repeated examination on the same day, with a tendency to increase in subsequent days (which may, however, be related to physiological changes in the portal flow). The interobserver agreement was always poor. Instrumentation variability [21] has also been ascertained, thus suggesting that follow-up examinations must be carried out on the same equipment and with the same transducer and angle.

These data, if confirmed, may raise some criticism concerning the reliability of flow volumes measured by Doppler method. At present it is reasonable to suppose that the Doppler spectrum reflects the actual blood flow in the portal vein, although the absolute values expressed in terms of millimeters per minute may not correspond to the real flow volumes. Changes in mean velocity and flow volume assessed by Doppler flowmetry in the same subject under different conditions are more acceptable [1], since possible sources of errors in measuring the absolute values are expected to affect different measurements in the same way. The method therefore seems suitable for in vivo monitoring of acute hemodynamic changes in the portal vein such as those induced by meal, hormones [2, 13], drugs, and other vasoactive substances.

Nevertheless, many papers dealing with quantitative measurements of flow in the portal vein have been published in recent years, and these agree that velocity is reduced, to a greater or lesser degree, in cirrhosis patients in comparison with healthy subjects (Fig. 9) [13, 24, 27, 36]. Data on portal flow volumes in liver cirrhosis are even more variable because the development of collateral pathways, which is different from case to case, greatly influences portal flow volume. Large splenorenal collaterals may reduce portal flow and even cause its reversal (Fig. 5) while a patent and dilated paraumbilical vein (Fig. 2) may explain high velocity and volume of portal flow. As regard the clinical meaning of these collaterals, Mostbeck et al. reported that a massive hepatofugal flow through a large paraumbilical vein may reduce the risk of variceal bleeding [25].

We have demonstrated [13] that 60 min after a standard meal a significant increase occurs in mean caliber, mean velocity, and flow volume in the portal vein of healthy subjects and in patients with chronic active hepatitis but not in patients with liver cirrhosis and portal hypertension. This behavior is probably related to increased intrahepatic resistance, to the hypertensive state in the splanchnic venous bed preventing further increase in portal flow, and to the diversion of blood flow by portosystemic collaterals.

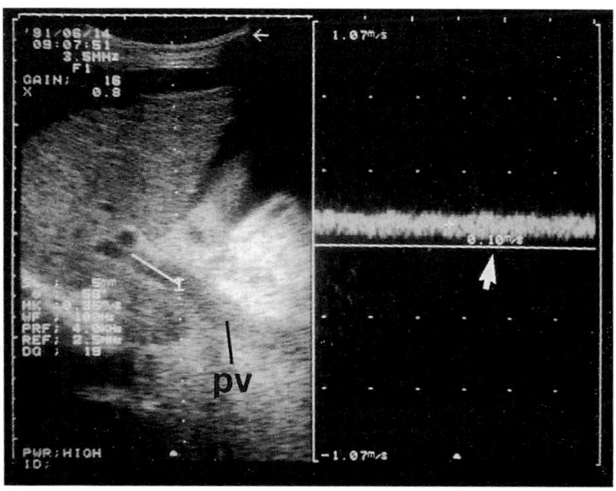

Fig. 9. Doppler flowmetry of the portal vein *(pv)* in patient with decompensated liver cirrhosis. The estimated mean velocity of flow is 10 cm/s *(arrow)*. Right intercostal scan

Doppler flowmetry is expected to make an important contribution in the evaluation of drug treatment of portal hypertension. This method may be useful in understanding the mechanism of the pharmacological effect, detecting nonresponders, and establishing the dosage and efficacy of new drugs. The drugs currently used in acute and chronic treatment of portal hypertension may be classified generally as vasoconstrictors or vasodilators [17], and the net effect of the reduction in portal pressure is reached through different mechanisms. In the case of blood flow reduction, this can be investigated by Doppler ultrasound, as has been demonstrated in recent years [20, 26, 37].

Since portal blood flow is strictly related to portal vascular resistance and portal pressure, and the change in any of these parameters influences the others, we think that Doppler findings on flow in the portal vein and the superior mesenteric, splenic, and hepatic arteries will help in elucidating the mechanism of action of any drug effective on portal pressure. Furthermore, the effect of the drug on collateral circulation, and particularly in the left gastric vein, can be investigated by Doppler ultrasound in selected patients with large and straight collaterals [14]. Transesophageal probes will also allow carefull evaluation of hemodynamic changes induced by the drug at the level of the azygos vein and esophagogastric varices [33]. These possibilities represent major advances for evaluation of the efficacy of a pharmacological treatment of portal hypertension, since the effect of any vasoactive drug on systemic circulation and portal pressure may not be strictly proportional to the effect on the collateral circulation or variceal pressure.

References

1. Barbara L (1990) The value of Doppler US in the study of hepatic hemodynamics. Consensus conference, Bologna, 12 Sep 1989. J Hepatol 10: 353–355
2. Bolondi L, Gaiani S, Li Bassi S, Casanova P, Zironi G, Barbara L (1990) Effect of secretin on portal venous flow. Gut 31: 1306–1310
3. Bolondi L, Li Bassi S, Gaiani S et al. (1991) Liver cirrhosis: changes of Doppler waveform of hepatic veins. Radiology 178: 513–516
4. Bolondi L, Gaiani S, Li Bassi S, Zironi G, Bonino F, Brunetto M, Barbara L (1991) Diagnosis of Budd-Chiari syndrome by pulsed Doppler ultrasound. Gastroenterology 100: 1324–1331
5. Bosch J, Groszmann RJ (1984) Measurement of the azygos venous blood flow by a continuous thermodilution technique. An index of blood flow through gastroesophageal collaterals in cirrhosis. Hepatology 4: 424–429
6. Burcharth F, Aagaard J (1988) Total hepatofugal portal flow in cirrhosis demonstrated by hepatic portography. ROFO 148/1: 47–49
7. Burchell AR, Moreno AH, Panke WF, Rousselot LM (1965) Some limitations of splenic portography. I. Incidence, hemodinamic and surgical implications of the nonvisualized portal vein. Ann Surg 162: 981–995
8. Burns P (1987) Doppler flowmetry and portal hypertension. Gastroenterology 92: 824–826
9. Caesar J, Shaldon S, Chiandussi L et al. (1961) The use of indocyanin green in the measurement of hepatic blood flow and as a test of hepatic function. Clin Sci 21: 43–57

10. Darnault P, Bretagne JF, Fournier V, Raoul J (1989) Splenic hemodynamic assessment in patients with liver cirrhosis and hypersplenism. Gastroenterology 96: A589
11. Dauzat M, Pomier Layrargues G (1989) Portal vein blood flow measurements using pulsed Doppler and electromagnetic flometry in dogs: a comparative study. Gastroenterology 96: 913–919
12. Foster DN, Herlinger H, Miloszewski KJA et al. (1978) Hepatofugal portal blood flow in hepatic cirrhosis. Ann Surg 187: 179–182
13. Gaiani S, Bolondi L, Li Bassi S, Santi V, Zironi G, Barbara L (1989) Effect of meal on portal hemodynamics in healthy humans and in patients with chronic liver disease. Hepatology 9: 815–819
14. Gaiani S, Bolondi L, Fenyves D, Zironi G, Rigamonti A, Barbara L (1991) Effect of propranolol on portosystemic collateral circulation in patients with liver cirrhosis. Hepatology 14: 824–829
15. Gaiani S, Bolondi L, Li Bassi S, Zironi G, Siringo S, Barbara L (1991) Prevalence of spontaneous hepatofugal flow in liver cirrhosis. Clinical and endoscopic correlation in 228 patients. Gastroenterology 100: 160–167
16. Gill RW (1979) Pulsed Doppler with B-mode imaging for quantitative blood flow measurement. Ultrasound Med Biol 5: 223–235
17. Groszmann RJ (1987) Drug therapy of portal hypertension. AJR Am J Roentgenol 82: 107–113
18. Huet PM, Lavoie P, Viallet A (1973) Simultaneous estimation of hepatic and portal blood flows by an indicator dilution technique. J Lab Clin Med 83: 836–846
19. Hunt AH, Whittard BR (1954) Thrombosis of the portal vein in cirrhosis hepatis. Lancet i: 281–284
20. Kawasaki T, Moriyasu F, Kimuura T et al. (1988) Study of the portal hemodynamic changes induced by dobutamine using an ultrasonic Doppler duplex system. J Ultrasound Med 7: S268
21. Kimme-Smith C, Hussain R, Duerinckx A, Tessler F, Grant E (1988) Reproducibility of Doppler abdominal flow rates: instrumentation variability. J Ultrasound Med 7: A1242
22. Longley DG, Skolnick ML, Sheahan DG (1988) Acute allograft rejection in liver transplant recipients: lack of correlation with loss of hepatic artery distolic flow. Radiology 169: 417–420
23. Moreno AH, Burchell AR, Rousselot LM, Panke WF, Slafsky SF, Burke JH (1967) Portal blood flow in cirrhosis of the liver. J Clin Invest 46: 436–445
24. Moriyasu F, Nishida O, Ban N et al. (1986) Measurement of portal vascular resistance in patients with portal hypertension. Gastroenterology 90: 710–717
25. Mostbeck GH, Wittich GR, Herold C, Vergesslich KA, Walter RM, Frotz S, Sommer G (1989) Hemodynamic significance of the paraumbilical vein in portal hypertension: assessment with duplex US. Radiology 170: 339–342
26. Navasa M, Bosch J, Reichen J et al. (1988) Effects of verapamil on hepatic and systemic hemodynamics and liver function in patients with cirrhosis and portal hypertension. Hepatology 8: 850–854
27. Ohnishi K, Saito M, Nakayama T et al. (1985) Portal venous hemodynamic in chronic liver disease: effects of posture change and exercise. Radiology 155: 757–761
28. Okuda K, Moriyama M, Yasumoto M et al. (1973) Roentgenologic demonstration of spontaneous reversal of portal blood flow in cirrhosis and hepatocellular carcinoma. AJR Am J Roentgenol 119: 419–428
29. Okuda K, Ohnishi K, Kimura K et al. (1985) Incidence of portal vein thrombosis in liver cirrhosis. An angiographic study in 708 patients. Gastroenterology 89: 279–286
30. Price JB, Voorhees AB Jr, Britton RC (1967) Operative hemodynamic study in portal hypertension. Significance and limitations. Arch Surg 95: 843–851
31. Rector WG, Hoefs JC, Hossack KF et al. (1988) Hepatofugal portal flow in cirrhosis: observations on hepatic hemodynamics and the nature of the arterioportal communications. Hepatology 8: 16–20

32. Sabbà C, Weltin G, Cicchetti DV et al. (1990) Observer variability in echo-Doppler measurements of portal flow in cirrhotic patients and in normal volunteers. Gastroenterology 98: 1603–1611
33. Sukigara M, Ohata M, Komazaki T, Matsumoto T, Omoto R (1988) The effect of propanolol on the venous flow in the azygos vein, intercostal vein and the esophagogastric varices. An evaluation using transesophageal real-time two-dimensional Doppler echography. J Ultrasound Med 7: S 190
34. Taylor KJW, Burns PN, Woodcock JP et al. (1985) Blood flow in deep abdominal and pelvic vessels: ultrasonic pulsed Doppler analysis. Radiology 154: 487–493
35. Taylor KJW, Morse SS, Weltin GG, Riely CA, Flye MW (1986) Liver transplant recipients: portable Duplex US with correlative angiography. Radiology 159: 357–363
36. Zoli M, Marchesini G, Cordiani MR et al. (1986)Echo-Doppler measurement of splanchnic blood flow in control and in cirrhotic subjects. J Clin Ultrasound 14: 429–435
37. Zoli M, Marchesini G, Brunori A, Cordiani MR, Pisi E (1986) Portal venous flow in response to acute β-blocker and vasodilatatory treatment in patients with liver cirrhosis. Hepatology 6: 1248–1251

Color Doppler Endosonography in the Study of Portal Hypertension

L. Bolondi, S. Gaiani, G. Zironi, F. Fornari, S. Siringo, and L. Barbara

Introduction

Endosonography provides significant additional information in the study of the esophageal and gastric wall [3, 13, 17, 28] and of extraluminal structures [13, 24, 25]. In the study of the esophagus the technique provides important data for the diagnosis and staging of esophageal carcinoma and for the morphological evaluation of varices and periesophageal collaterals. In portal hypertension patients the technique supplies new data for the assessment of hypertensive gastropathy [9].

The recent development of duplex Doppler endosonographic transducers, combining real-time imaging with Doppler flowmetry, has opened new possibilities, particularly in the field of cardiology [16], where these methods have replaced in most cases the invasive hemodynamic techniques. Doppler evaluation of blood flow in the esophageal varices was previously obtained by blind transducers [20, 21]. These studies emphasized the hemodynamic role of the perforating veins connecting the esophageal varices to the periesophageal veins and demonstrated that blood flow in esophageal varices is not always cephalad and may sometimes run toward the stomach. In these studies, however, the absence of ultrasonographic imaging made it difficult to identify the vessels and obviously prevented the assessment of morphological parameters, such as the caliber of the vessel itself. The last generation of these devices are also equipped with fiberoptic endoscopes, thus allowing one to combine endoscopic assessment of varices with ultrasonography and Doppler flowmetry. Using this technique [26, 27] new hemodynamic data concerning esophageal and gastric varices, periesophageal collaterals, and the azygos vein have recently been collected.

Measurement of Azygos Vein Blood Flow by Thermodilution Technique

It is known that gastroesophageal collaterals drain mainly into the superior vena cava through the azygos venous system. The measurement of blood flow in this vein may therefore represent useful index of collateral hepatofugal flow in patients with portal hypertension. The thermodilution technique of the catheterized azygos vein is usually performed for this purpose [4];

however, since this is invasive and cumbersome, it is reserved only to specialized laboratories. This procedure demonstrated a significant increase in azygos venous flow in patients with portal hypertension in comparison with controls, and a direct correlation of azygos venous flow with portal pressure and size of esophageal varices [5]. Despite a correlation of azygos flow with the amount of previous bleeding, the method seems unable to predict the risk of hemorrhage.

Apart from the measurement of azygos flow in basal condition, the technique allows quantification of flow changes following instrumental and pharmacological treatment of portal hypertension. It has been demonstrated that azygos flow significantly decreases after portosystemic shunt operation, Sengstaken-Blakemore tamponade [5], and endoscopic sclerotherapy [18]. The technique found its major applications in the evaluation of pharmacological agents such as vasopressin [23], furosemide [12], ketanserin [15], somatostatin [7], β-blockers [5, 8], isosorbide-5-mononitrate [22], metoclopramide, and domperidone [19].

The observation that some drugs induce similar reduction in portal pressure but different changes in azygos vein blood flow supports the hypothesis that pharmacological agents may be effective on portocollateral resistance, and consequently the evaluation of the effect of drugs by the hepatic vein catheterization and pressure measurement may only partially reflect the hemodynamic activity of the drug itself. Regarding this point, it has been observed that in patients with normal or relatively high portal pressure, large pressure changes correspond to small changes in the azygos venous flow. On the other hand, in patients with high portal pressure, small pressure changes correspond to large variation in the azygos venous flow. This suggests that the measure of azygos venous flow may be more sensitive than that of portal pressure for assessing the effect of therapy in portal hypertensive patients. In addition, relatively unknown are the effects on azygos venous flow of a particular hemodynamic pattern, such as the reversal of portal venous flow, which may be relatively frequent in these patients [14].

Color Doppler Endosonography: Personal Experience

Instrumentation and Technique of Examination

We utilized the real-time ultrasonographic equipment AU 590 (Esaote-Hitachi) provided by pulsed Doppler and color flow mapping. The 7.5-MHz convex array transducer, with an angle of view of 100°, is positioned longitudinally on the tip of the fibroscope Pentax FG32UA. The nonflexible tip of the transducer is 4 cm long. The ultrasonic beam is directed laterally to the tip, and the scanning plane is longitudinal to the axis of the endoscope. This makes the images obtained by this equipment substantially different from those obtained by conventional endosonographic rotating transducers, which provide transverse axial scans extended up to 360° [2]. A small balloon distended by deaired water may be used to facilitate the contact with esophageal wall and the focusing of superficially located lesions. The examination is carried out with the patients lying on left side decubitus, after a premedication with 5 mg joscin *N*-butylbromure and local anesthesia with lidocaine.

During the first part of the examination the endoscopic view allows one to assess the presence, location, and size of varices, guiding the subsequent ultrasonographic and Doppler examination. Periesophageal collateral vessels are detected by rotating the endoscopic probe within the distal tract of the

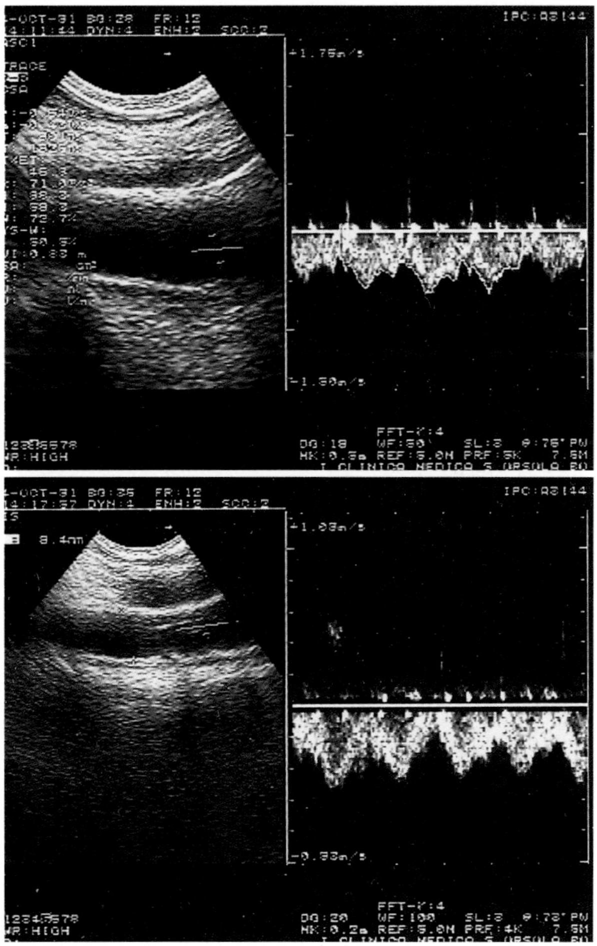

Fig. 1. The longitudinal tract of the azygos vein visualized by 7.5-MHz endoscopic convex array at two different levels: distal *(above)* and proximal *(below)*. The Doppler spectral analysis in both cases shows a phasic waveform with a maximal flow velocity close to 50 cm/s in the distal tract

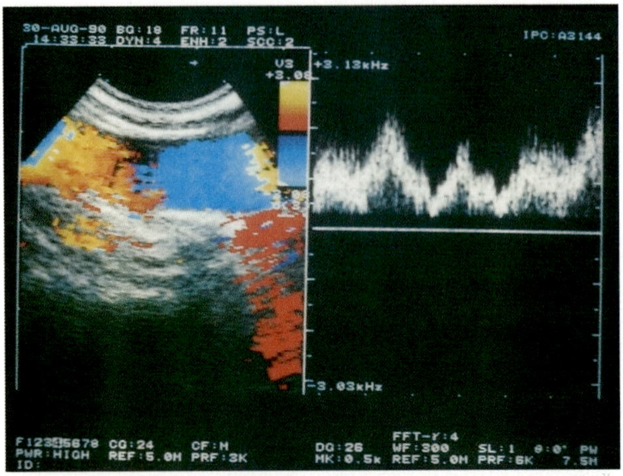

Fig. 2. Color Doppler imaging of the longitudinal tract of the azygos vein. Also in this case the Doppler spectral analysis shows a phasic waveform, similar to that occurring in the vena cava

esophagus. These appear as anechoic longitudinal channels with a tortuous course. Pulsed Doppler evaluation of esophageal varices and periesophageal veins may be difficult because of their irregular and winding course. However, a rough assessment of direction of flow and maximal flow velocity (V_{max}) may be obtained in most cases. Color flow mapping allows easy detection of the direction of flow and the presence of turbulence. The azygos vein is visualized by positioning the transducer close to the posterior esophageal wall at a distance of about 20–25 cm from the mouth. Starting from the image of the thoracic aorta the probe is turned to the left until the vein is identified (Figs. 1, 2). The caliber of the azygos vein is measured at two different levels: in the lower tract and in the curving distal tract, before the confluence with the inferior vena cava.

The Doppler study is performed both in the proximal (lower) and in the distal (upper) curving tract, where the angle of insonation is always optimal (20°–50°). The estimate of flow obtained at this level is of particular importance because it reflects the whole blood flow of the azygos venous system running into the inferior vena cava. In our study we measured the maximal velocity of flow in the proximal and the distal (curving) tract of the vein using angles of insonation ranging from 20° to 50° and calculating, by special software of the instrument, the mean value of V_{max} for periods of 4–6 s.

Patients

The present study was performed in 22 cirrhotic patients (7 with hepatocellular carcinoma). Fifteen of these patients had esophageal varices detected at endoscopy. These varices were classified, on the basis of the JRSPH rules [1], as grade I in eight cases, grade II in five cases, and grade III in two cases. In all patients we measured the vessel caliber and the V_{max} at the proximal and distal tract of the azygos vein and assessed the presence of periesophageal varices.

Results

The endosonographic visualization of esophageal varices was difficult in most cases because of the compression of the probe itself on the vessels and the poor ultrasonographic focusing of structures immediately close to the probe.

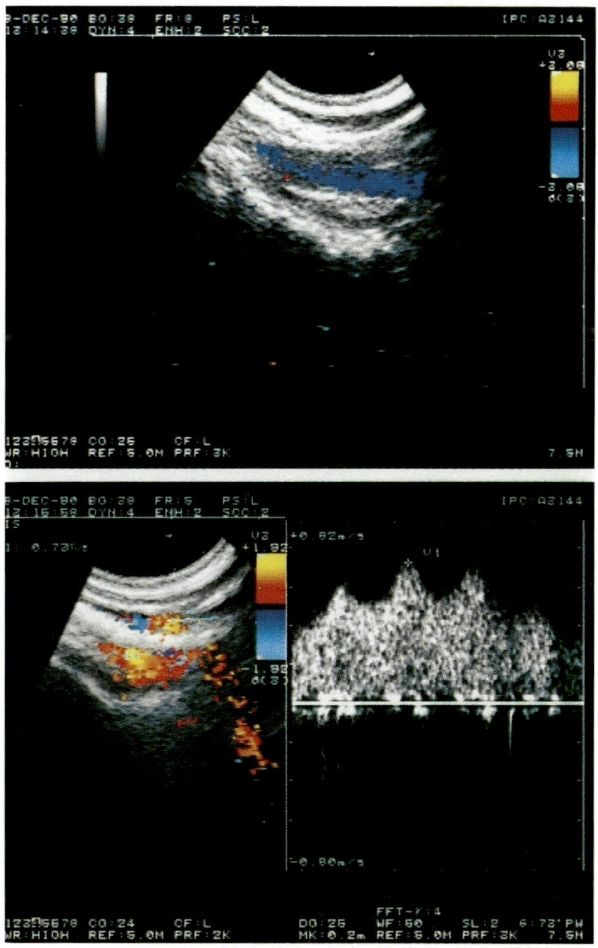

Fig. 3. Color Doppler imaging of esophageal varices and periesophageal vessels. *Below,* the spectral analysis, performed in a superficial varice, shows a high frequency, turbulent Doppler trace, with a peak velocity of 73 cm/s

It was obtained in 11 of 15 cases (73.3 %); complete visualization of varices along their course was achieved in only 4 cases. The Doppler flowmetry showed a wide range of velocities (25–90 cm/s) with marked turbulence (Fig. 3).

The azygos vein and its confluence into the inferior vena cava was detectable in all patients. The length of the visualized tract ranged from 4 to 7 cm. The caliber of the vein was 7.4±2.2 mm in the proximal tract and 9.4±3.2 mm in the distal tract. We observed a significant difference in both proximal and distal calibers of the azygos vein between patients with and those without varices (proximal tract: 8.1±2.2 mm versus 6.1±1.8 mm, $p < 0.05$; distal tract: 10.4±3.1 mm versus 8.9±2.2 mm, $p < 0.01$). In 20 out of 22 patients we observed a phasic Doppler waveform (Figs. 1, 2, 4), similar to that of the inferior vena cava, while in two patients the flow profile was more continuous and flat (Fig. 5). The V_{max} was 67±34 cm/s in the proximal tract and 54±26 cm/s in the distal arcuate tract. The values of V_{max} tended to be higher, without reaching statistical significance, in patients with esophageal varices.

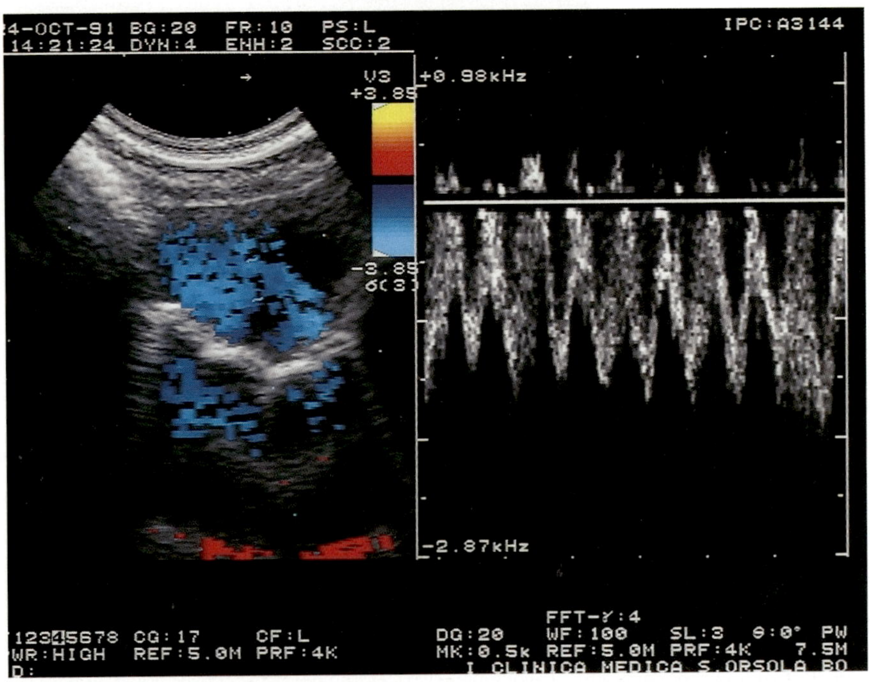

Fig. 4. Color Doppler imaging of the distal curving tract of the azygos vein, with a phasic pattern upon Doppler spectral analysis

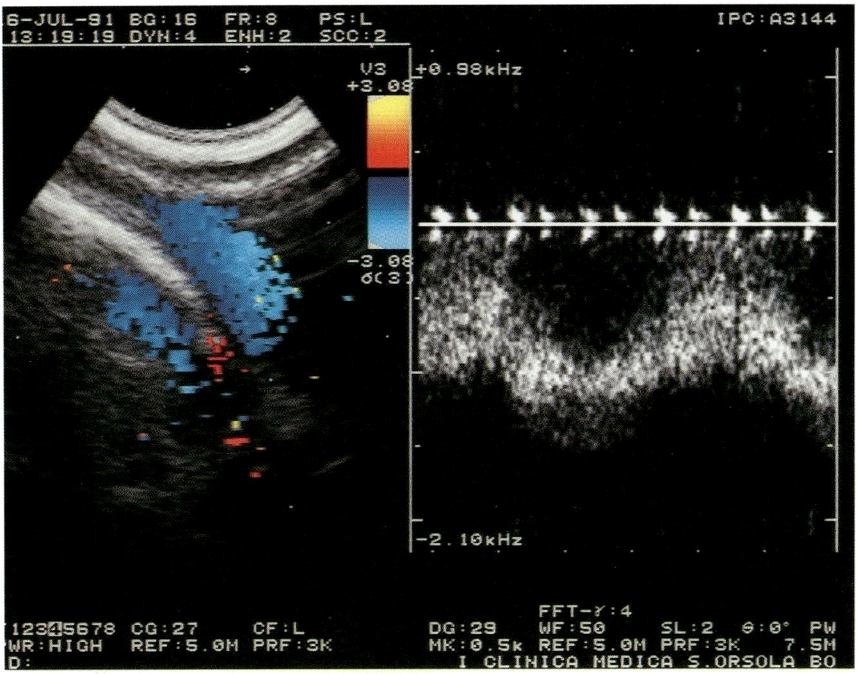

Fig. 5. Color Doppler imaging of the distal tract of the azygos vein. In this case the waveform appears less phasic than in the cases represented in Figs. 1 and 2

Discussion

The utility of endosonography [10, 11] and Doppler endosonography [26, 27] in the study of portal hypertension has been outlined in recent papers. In particular it has been demonstrated that Doppler endosonography can provide a reliable estimate of azygos blood flow which correlates with thermodilution measurements [26, 27].

In our study we utilized an instrumentation combining the endoscopic view and the ultrasonographic image together with color Doppler and pulsed Doppler flowmetry. This association substantially improves the technique of examination, particularly for the identification of varices and the subsequent positioning of the probe into the esophageal lumen. Another major advantage of this instrument in comparison with the rotating transducers previously utilized in endosonography is the possibility of connecting the probe to the new, commercially available sophisticated ultrasound equipment with color and pulsed Doppler technology. With this new generation of endoscopic transducers, a special machine is no longer required for endoscopic ultrasonography. The endoscopic transducer can therefore be considered as an accessory device of the conventional ultrasound equipment to be utilized in selected patients where particular hemodynamic information is needed.

This preliminary study assessed the feasibility of the Doppler flowmetry in the azygos vein, which represents a critical point in the complex hemodynamics of portal hypertension. We have demonstrated that this vessel is easily detectable by this Doppler endosonographic instrumentation, which is able to give information regarding the flow profile and the velocity and turbulence in the azygos vein. Further studies, correlating Doppler endosonography with endoscopy, Doppler flowmetry of the portal vein, and clinical data, are required to clarify the diagnostic and prognostic potential of this new method.

References

1. Beppu K, Inokuchi K, Koyanagi N et al. (1981) Prediction of variceal hemorrhage by esophageal endoscopy. Gastrointest Endosc 27: 213–218
2. Bolondi L, Caletti GC, Barbara L (1989) Endoscopic sonography of the esophagus. In: Formage BD (ed) Endosonography. Kluwer, Dordrecht, pp 25–34
3. Bolondi L, Casanova P, Caletti GC, Grigioni W, Zani L, Barbara L (1987) Primary gastric limphoma versus gastric carcinoma: endoscopic US evaluation
4. Bosch J, Groszmann RJ (1984) Measurement of the azygos blood flow by a continuous thermodilution technique. An index of blood flow through gastroesophageal collaterals in cirrhosis. Hepatology 4: 424–429
5. Bosch J, Mastai R, Kravetz D et al. (1984) Effects of propranolol on azygos venous blood flow and hepatic and systemic hemodynamics in cirrhosis. Hepatology 4: 1200–1205
6. Bosch J, Mastai R, Kravetz D, Bruix J, Rigau J, Rodés J (1985) Measurement of azygos venous blood flow in the evaluation of portal hypertension in patients with cirrhosis. Clinical and hemodynamic correlations in 100 patients. J Hepatol 1: 125–139
7. Bosch J, Kravetz D, Mastai R et al. (1983) Azygos venous blood flow in cirrhosis. Effect of balloon tamponade, vasopressin, somatostatin and propranolol. Hepatology 3: 855
8. Cales P, Braillon J, Jiron M et al. (1985) Superior portosystemic collateral circulation estimated by azygos blood flow in patients with cirrhosis. J Hepatol 1: 37–46
9. Caletti GC, Bolondi L, Zani L, Brocchi E, Guizzardi G, Barbara L (1986) Detection of portal hypertension and esophageal varices by means of endoscopic ultrasonography. Scand J Gastroenterol Suppl 21: 74–77
10. Caletti GC, Brocchi E, Zani L, Bolondi L, Festi D, Casanova P, Barbara L (1989) Endosonography (EUT) in portal hypertension. In: Dancygier H, Classen M (eds) Proceedings of the 5th symposium on endoscopic ultrasonography, Munich, 10–11 July 1987. Demeter, Graefelfing, pp 46–49
11. Caletti GC, Brocchi E, Baraldini M, Ferrari A, Gibilaro M, Barbara L (1990) Assessment of portal hypertension by endoscopic ultrasonography. Gastrointest Endosc 36: S21 – S27
12. Cereda JM, Roulot D, Braillon A, Moreau R, Koshy A, Lebrec D (1989) Reduction of portal pressure by acute administration of furosemide in patients with alcoholic cirrhosis. J Hepatol 9: 246–251
13. Di Magno EP, Regan PT, Clain JE, James EM, Buxton JL (1982) Human endoscopic ultrasonography. Gastroenterology 83: 824–829
14. Gaiani S, Bolondi L, LiBassi S, Zironi G, Siringo S, Barbara L (1991) Prevalence of spontaneous hepatofugal portal flow in liver cirrhosis. Clinical and endoscopic correlation in 228 patients. Gastroenterology 100: 160–167

15. Hadengue A, Lee SS, Moreau R, Braillon A, Lebrec D (1987) Beneficial hemodynamic effects of ketanserin in patients with cirrhosis: possible role of serotonergic mechanisms in portal hypertension. Hepatology 7: 644–647
16. Hanrath P, Schluter M, Langerstein BA et al. (1983) Detection of ostium secundum atrial septal defects by transesophageal cross-sectional echocardiography. Br Heart J 49: 350–358
17. Lux G, Heyder N, Lutz H, Demling L (1982) Endoscopic ultrasonography. Technique, orientation and diagnostic possibilities. Endoscopy 14: 220–225
18. Mastai R, Bosch J, Bordas JM et al. (1985) Efecto de la esclerosis de varices esofagicas sobre el flujo sanguineo de la vena acigos en pacientes con hipertension portal. Gastroenterol Hepatol 8: 174
19. Mastai R, Grande L, Bosch J et al. (1986)Effects of metoclopramide and domperidone on azygos venous blood flow in patients with cirrhosis and portal hypertension. Hepatology 6: 1244–1247
20. McCormack TT, Johnson AG et al. (1983) Doppler ultrasound probe for assessment of blood flow in oesophageal varices. Lancet i: 677–678
21. McCormack TT, Rose JD, Smith PM, Johnson AG (1983) Perforating veins and blood flow in oesophageal varices. Lancet i: 1442–1444
22. Navasa M, Chesta J, Bosch J, Rodés J (1989) Reduction of portal pressure by isosorbide-5-mononitrate in patients with cirrhosis. Gastroenterology 96: 1110–1118
23. Rector WG, Hossack KF (1989) Vasopressin and vasopressin plus nitroglycerin for portal hypertension. Effects on systemic and splanchnic hemodynamics and coronary blood flow. J Hepatol 8: 308–315
24. Rifkin MD, Gordon SJ, Goldberg BB (1984) Sonographic examination of the mediastinum and upper abdomen by fiberoptic gastroscope. Radiology 151: 175–180
25. Strohm WD, Kurtz W, Hagenmuller F, Classen M (1984) Diagnostic efficacy of endoscopic ultrasound tomography in pancreatic cancer and cholestasis. Scand J Gastroenterol 19: 18–23
26. Sukigara M, Komazaki T, Yamazaki T et al. (1987) Color flow mapping of the esophageal varices and vessels in and around the liver with real-time two-dimensional Doppler echography. Clin Radiol 38: 487–494
27. Sukigara M, Shimoji K, Ohata M et al. (1988) Effects of propranolol and nitroglycerin on cephalad collateral venous flow in patients with cirrhosis: evaluation using transesophageal real-time two-dimensional Doppler echography. Am J Gastroenterol 83: 1248–1254
28. Tanaka Y, Yasuda K, Aibe T, Fuji T, Kawai K (1984) Anatomical and pathological aspects in ultrasonic endoscopy for G.I. tract. Scand J Gastroenterol Suppl 19: 43–50

Cystogastric Catheter Drainage of Pancreatic Collections of Fluid Under Endoscopic/Ultrasonographic Guidance

N. Heyder, E. Günter, and E. G. Hahn

Introduction

In 1985 Hancke published a report on cystogastrostomy using a double-pigtail catheter as an alternative to surgical drainage of pseudocysts. With the aim of testing the technique we carried out a prospective study between 1986 and 1991 in 39 patients with 40 pancreatic collections of fluid. The object of the study was to identify those collections of fluid that would be suitable for cystogastric drainage.

As described elsewhere [1, 2], in *cystogastric drainage,* after prior localization of the cyst, a polyethylene catheter having an outside diameter of 2.8 mm is introduced percutaneously into the stomach and under ultrasonographic control is advanced through the posterior wall of the stomach into the cyst. The catheter is curled at both ends (double-pigtail catheter) and for introduction is passed over a 22-cm-long cannula. A tube (pusher) fitted over the cannula proximal to the catheter keeps the latter in the desired position while the cannula is being removed. As soon as the cannula has been withdrawn, the distal end of the catheter curls up within the cyst and the proximal end within the stomach, thus preventing dislodgement (Fig. 1). When in place, the length of the catheter is 8 cm. Removal is effected via the endoscope using the polypectomy loop.

In *percutaneous drainage,* a pigtail catheter is inserted percutaneously into the cyst, and the latter is drained until no further fluid issues [3]. In *pure endoscopic gastrocystostomy* or *duodenocystostomy,* the gastric or duodenal wall, together with the wall of the cyst is opened via the endoscope with the aid of the electrotome, and (also via the endoscope) a catheter is inserted into the cyst, the contents of which then drain into the stomach or duodenum, respectively [4, 5]. With these procedures, it is necessary for the pseudocyst to be pressing up against the wall of the stomach or the duodenum [5]. In the case of surgical drainage of the cyst, the latter is anastomosed with the stomach or duodenum, but preferentially with a loop of the jejunum via a laparotomy. With this procedure, the cyst must be mature enough for its wall to retain the suture.

The various pancreatic collections of fluid require a number of different therapeutic approaches. Persistent pancreatic ascites occurs in the presence of a leakage in the pancreatic duct system. In such a case, the sole treatment is surgical. Chronic pancreatic cysts, as defined below, need to be treated only if

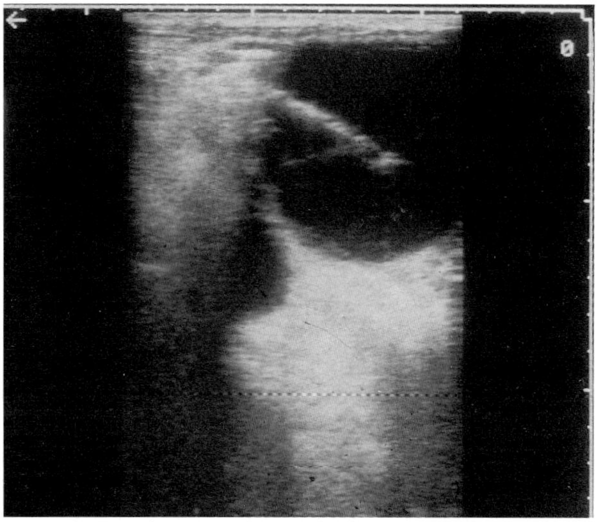

Fig. 1. Catheter during insertion from the stomach into the pseudocyst

they give rise to such complications as obstruction of the common bile duct. In most cases, the wall is too tough to permit penetration by the drainage catheter, so that they require a surgical or endoscopic-operative approach. The decision as to whether acute necroses require conservative or surgical treatment depends upon the course of the disease. Postacute pseudocysts clear up spontaneously in 40 % – 60 % of cases [6, 7]. Persistent postacute pseudocysts should be treated, since apart from pain a sensation of fullness and obstruction of the common bile duct, stomach, or duodenum they can also give rise to life-threatening complications such as abscesses and erosion of major blood vessels [6, 8].

Patients and Prospective Protocol

A total of 30 men and 9 women aged between 24 and 81 years (mean 42.6) were admitted to the study. One patient with a recurrence was treated twice, and the second drainage procedure was successful.

Differentiation of pancreatic collections of fluid as described below was necessary for both the planning of the study and the evaluation of the results. The designation "pancreatic collections of fluid" served as a collective term. We employed the term "acute necrosis" to describe circumscribed collections of fluid not older than 6 weeks and lacking a definable wall. The term "postacute pseudocyst" was employed to describe circumscribed collections of fluid of pancreatic origin with a distinct wall and an age of more than 6 weeks. We did not differentiate between postacute pseudocysts arising in a chronically inflamed and those found in a previously healthy pancreas. We used the expression "chronic pseudocyst" to describe collections of fluid having a diameter of up to 3 cm, a thick wall, and an age of more than 6 months. The term "pancreatic ascites" was used to designate free fluid with an amylase content of more 100 times that of the normal serum level.

In all 40 patients chronic, parasitic, congenital, and neoplastic pancreatic cysts, fistulae, and pancreatic ascites were considered exclusion criteria. It was intended that the experience gained with patients 1–20 should, where applicable, be applied to patients 21–40 with the aim of establishing whether additional exclusion criteria might improve the success rate. In the first five patients the procedure was carried out under insufflation anesthesia, thereafter under only local anesthesia (5–10 ml procaine, Novocain, 2%), with pain/sedation prophylaxis with 5 mg diazepam and 50 mg pethidine. Beginning with the third patient a 3-day antibiotic cover with imipenem 3 × 500 mg and tobramycin 2 × 80 mg, begun on the morning of the day of drainage, was administered prophylactically.

We analyzed the cyst in terms of age, maximum diameter, content (amylase, lipase, bacteriology), and emptying time. One week prior to drainage, on the evening of the day of drainage, and on the day after drainage we registered the temperature, leukocyte count, and serum amylase.

Follow-up examinations after placement of the drain on days 1 and 3, months 1, 3, 6, and 12 included ultrasound and serum amylase determination. Follow-up examinations after removal of the drain on day 1, months 1, 3, and 6 did likewise.

Results

The 40 pancreatic collections of fluid revealed 4 instances of necrosis and 36 of postacute cyst. The diameter ranged from 4.5 to 20 cm (mean 10.5) and the age from 2 weeks and 20 months. Amylase levels were 11 000–167 000 μ/l (mean 45 000; normal serum range 1–110 U/l) and lipase 40 000–5 600 000 μ/l (mean 873 000; normal serum range 1–190 U/l).

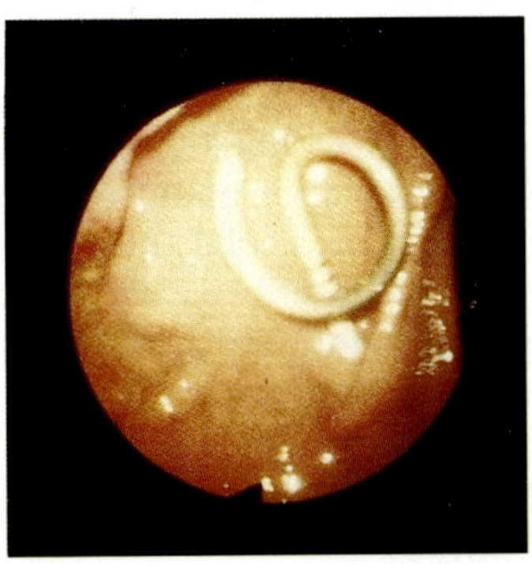

Fig. 2. Endoscopic aspect of the curled end of the catheter in the stomach. The other end of the catheter is curled in the cyst in the same way

The maximum diameter of the cyst, together with serum amylase and serum lipase levels, was determined immediately prior to and on the first and third days after placement of the catheter. Prior to drainage (Fig. 2) the maximum diameter varied between 4.5 and 20 cm (mean 10.5 cm) and on the first day following placement of the drain (Fig. 3) between 0 to 12.5 cm (mean 2.8 cm). Twenty-two patients had elevated serum amylase prior to the

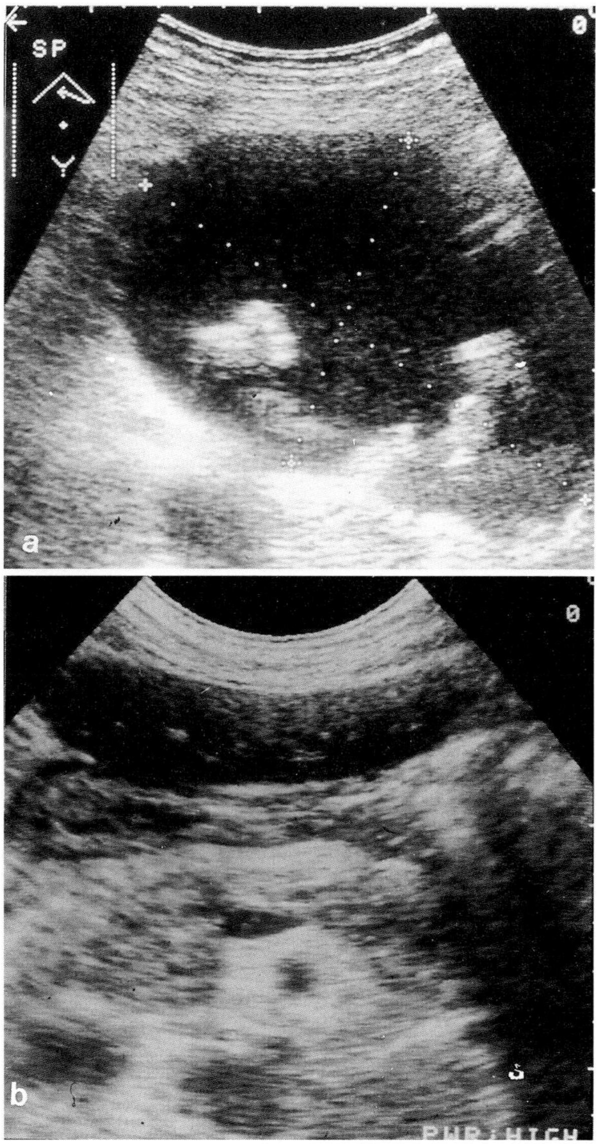

Fig. 3 a, b. Pancreatic pseudocyst. **a** Before cystogastric drainage. **b** Three days after cystogastric drainage

procedure. In 20 patients (91 %) serum amylase dropped on average from 419 to 290 U/l; in two patients (9 %) it rose from 132 to 409 U/l and from 155 to 308 U/l, respectively. Of the two patients with increasing amylase levels, one had a fresh necrosis. In the second, the amylase level decreased again to its initial value on the third day but fluctuated in the following months between 160 and 250 U/l. In this patient, the pseudocyst was completely evacuated after 4 weeks. In 32 patients, complete drainage occurred, in 21 (66 %) of these within 24 h. The longest time to complete evacuation was 8 weeks.

Indwelling times for the catheter were determined arbitrarily and were between 2 and 12 months, with a mean of 5.3 months. Puncture was considered successful when it led to a permanent diminution in the size of the cyst, with a maximum diameter of residual fluid of 2 cm.

Causes of the failure of cystogastric drainage in 9 of the first 20 patients were: cyst immaturity, preexisting infection, recurrence, BII stomach, cyst too small, and dislodgement (catheter too short). Using these conditions as exclusion criteria in the second 20 patients led to an improvement in the success rate from 55 % (11/20) to 75 % (15/20). The failures of cystogastric drainage among patients 21–40 were caused by recurrence of the cyst and acute inflammation.

There was one case of bacterial infection and two of infection with *Candida albicans*. In the former, who had a 2-week-old infected necrosis and a preprocedure temperature of 38.6 °C, the temperature rose to 40.1 °C on the evening of the day of the drainage. Three other patients developed a temperature of up to 38.9 °C; these three included two in whom the intervention had been carried out without antibiotic cover. Under antibiotic treatment the temperature normalized within 3 days in both cases. The third patient had a 5-week old necrosis with preexisting *Candida albicans* infection and had to be sent for surgery after 1 week. The attempt at drainage had resulted in bacterial superinfection. Three patients with preexisting infections had to be submitted to surgery within 2 weeks after the procedure. Two patients with necroses were successfully treated with additional transcutaneous catheter drainage and thus spared surgery. In both, the cystogastric drainage catheter was withdrawn after 1 week. In all patients with necrosis and/or infection, the catheter was blocked at this time.

In 18 patients (45 %) we established an elevated leukocyte count of up to 23 000/mm^3 (mean 13 500) on the evening of the day of the drainage. These figures normalized again within 36 h in all patients with the exception of those with preexisting infection or necroses.

Complications. One of the two patients with prior *Candida albicans* infection became febrile after cystogastric drainage as a result of bacterial superinfection (2.5 %). Otherwise we observed no severe complications, in particular no recognizable hemorrhage, no perforation, and no fatal complications. All patients submitted to surgery survived the intervention.

Technical Problems. In four cases drainage failed for anatomical, puncture-related technical reasons, or for reasons associated with material failure. Two attempts to puncture a pancreatic head cyst measuring 4.5 cm in diameter failed, and the procedure was abandoned. In an additional case, the gastric stump remaining after a BII resection was too small and too high up in the abdominal cavity, so that puncture would have required an intercostal approach, which in turn would have greatly limited the freedom of movement of the puncture set. In the case of the third patient, we employed a catheter measuring only 6 cm in length, which was pulled out of the cyst by the peristaltic movements of the stomach. In another patient, the catheter broke in the middle after about 4 months, presumably due to material fatigue. The half that passed into the stomach was voided, unnoticed, with the feces, while the other half was removed surgically from a postacute pseudocyst that had shrunk and been completely replaced by scar tissue.

Discussion

The aim of the present study was to investigate whether and for what types of pancreatic collections of fluid endoscopy- and ultrasonography-guided cystogastric drainage could be suitably employed. In addition, we attempted to establish the earliest point in the natural history of the cyst at which the procedure could successfully be applied. Our results show that a precondition for the emptying of a pancreatic collection of fluid is a cicatricial wall, the shrinking of which raises the intracavitary pressure. In numerous cases, this results in rapid evacuation of the contents into the stomach and also explains why reflux in the reverse direction apparently does not occur – or at least only rarely. Since, however, reflux cannot be completely excluded, bacterial growth within the stomach should not be promoted by medication-induced reduction of gastric acid production.

The extremely high concentrations of amylase, lipase and elastase in the fluid draining from the cyst apparently prevents blockage of the catheter. This is not the case when the contents of the cyst are infected, when blockage of the catheter occurs despite the fact that infected cystic fluid also contains extremely high concentrations of amylase and lipase. These high enzyme concentrations in the fluid contained within the cyst would also explain hemorrhagic complications and perforation. Although endoscopic retrograde cholangiopancreatography (ERCP) reveals a connection between the pancreatic duct and cyst in only 44 % – 55 % of cases [4, 9], we also measured such high enzyme concentrations in postacute pseudocysts that were several months old. We therefore suspect some connection between the pancreatic duct system and persisting pseudocyst even when ERCP provides no evidence of such a connection. In 91 % of patients with elevated serum amylase, decompression of the pseudocyst resulted in a decrease in the serum level. The most likely explanation for this appears to be that the contents of the cyst pass into blood vessels adjacent to its wall; this would, however, mean that the enzyme concentration in the cyst should progressively decrease. The fact that this was not found to be the case can be explained only by assuming a connection to the ductal system.

The oldest of our cysts in which cystogastric drainage failed was 5 weeks; the youngest in which the procedure was successful was 8 weeks. A well developed, cicatricial cystic wall is also a precondition for surgical internal drainage (cystogastrostomy, cystoduodenostomy, cystojejunostomy). The time that it takes for this to develop is 6 weeks [10]. This means that the earliest time for endoscopy/ultrasonography-guided cystogastrostomy is probably between 6 and 8 weeks.

In three cases we had to remove the catheter before the cyst had completely drained, since excessive drinking had led to the development of new acute inflammatory processes and new pancreatic collections of fluid, and, as a foreign body, the catheter would have promoted the development of infections. This means that continued alcohol abuse modifies the indication for this form of drainage. We suspect that three patients began to drink more when, as a result of decompression of the cyst, pain largely disappeared.

Alternatives to endoscopy- and ultrasonography-guided cystogastric drainage are surgical cystoenterostomy, transcutaneous ultrasonography or computed tomography guided catheter drainage and endoscopic cystogastrostomy or cystoduodenostomy. In the absence of a uniform definition of the various pancreatic collections of fluid, a comparison of all the results and complication rates reported to date is problematical.

In the case of transcutaneous ultrasonography or computed tomography guided catheter drainage, the pseudocyst must either be in contact with the abdominal wall, or it must be possible to establish such contact by compression, since the catheter must not be allowed to pass through the bowel. In the case of external drainage, the presence of the catheter means that the patient is unlikely to be able to go to work. The advantages of internal drainage procedures in comparison with transcutaneous drainage are that the catheter does not hinder the patient, no loss of pancreatic secretion occurs, and the patient cannot remove the catheter himself. On the other hand, the success of transcutaneous drainage is less dependent on the intracavitary pressure than is the case with internal drainage since the contents of the cyst can also be aspirated. This also means that transcutaneous drainage can be carried out earlier than internal drainage. An additional advantage is that in the case of an infection irrigation, with or without the addition of antibiotics, can be performed. The success rate of transcutaneous catheter drainage is reported to be between 69% [11] and 90% [3]. Applying our exclusion criteria, cystogastric drainage achieves a success rate of 75%, which is thus comparable with that of transcutaneous drainage. The complication rate of external drainage is reported to be 29.6%, with a mortality rate of up to 14.8%.

In the case of endoscopic cystoenterostomy, a success rate of between 63.2% [4] (47.4% good and 15.8% satisfactory results) and 96% [5] for cystogastric drainage, and of 100% [5] for cystogastrostomy is reported [5].

The latter figures, however, do not take account of the recurrences, 9 % for cystoduodenostomy and 19 % for cystogastrostomy [5]. The complication rates associated with endoscopic cystoenterostomy are about 23.5 %. A single fatal complication due to hemorrhage has been reported [4]. In the case of endoscopic cystoenterostomy the cyst needs to be causing the stomach of duodenal wall to bulge. In the case of drainage guided by ultrasonography/endoscopy, this is not a requirement, although here too no blood vessels should be located in the puncture path. In case of doubt, an endoscopic ultrasonography should be performed to exclude the presence of any interposing vessels, preferentially with color coding. Using the purely endoscopic technique of cystoduodenostomy, small cysts in the head of the pancreas are technically easier to drain than with the procedure that we tested. However, we can see no principal difference between purely endoscopic and ultrasonography/endoscopy-guided internal catheter drainage. In comparable surgical case material, the success rates lie between 78 % [12] and 100 % [13], with a complication rate of 5.8 % [14].

In comparison with the surgical version, catheter drainage has the advantage of being less invasive. However, it is not suitable for a number of cases, including cysts arising from tumor-induced compression of the pancreatic duct, fistulae, hemosuccus pancreaticus, cysts into which there is bleeding, or sequesters, or cysts that cannot be drained with a catheter for anatomical reasons.

References

1. Hancke S, Henriksen FW (1985) Percutaneous pancreatic cysto-gastrostomy guided by ultrasound scanning and gastroscopy. Brit J Surg 72: 916–917
2. Heyder N, Flügel H, Domschke W (1988) Catheter drainage of pancreatic pseudocysts into the stomach. Endoscopy 20: 75–77
3. Van Sonnenberg E, Wittich GR, Casola G, Brannigan TC, Karnel F, Stabile BE, Varney RR, Christensen RR (1989) Percutaneous drainage of infected and noninfected pancreatic pseudocysts: experience in 101 cases. Radiology 170: 757–761
4. Sahel J, Bastid C, Pellat B, Schurgers P, Sarles H (1987) Endoscopic cystoduodenostomy of cysts of chronic calcifying pancreatitis. A report of 20 cases. Pancreas 2: 447–453
5. Cremer M, Deviere J, Engelholm L (1989) Endoscopic management of cysts and pseudocysts in chronic pancreatitis: long term follow-up after 7 years of experience. Gastrointest Endosc 35: 1–9
6. Bradley, EL, Clements JL jr, Gonzales AC (1979) The natural history of pancreatic pseudocysts: a unified concept of management. Amer J Surg 137: 135–141
7. Yeo CJ, Bastidas JA, Lynch-Nyhan A, Fishman EK, Zinner MJ, Cameron JL (1990) The natural history of pancreatic pseudocysts documented by computed tomography. Surg Gynecol Obstet 170: 411–417
8. Kiviluoto T, Kivisaari L, Kivilaakso E, Lempinen M (1989) Pseudocysts in chronic pancreatitis. Arch Surg 124: 240–243
9. Nealon WH, Townsend CM, Thompson JC (1989) Preoperative endoscopic retrograde cholangiopancreatography (ERCP) in patients with pancreatic pseudocysts associated with resolving acute and chronic pancreatitis. Ann Surg 209: 532–540
10. Warshaw AL, Rattner DW (1985) Timing of surgical drainage for pancreatic pseudocyst. Clinical and chemical criteria. Ann Surg 202: 720–724

11. Stanley JH, Gobien RP, Schabel SI, Andriole JG, Anderson MC, Smith RW (1988) Percutaneous drainage of pancreatic and peripancreatic fluid collections. Cardiovasc Intervent Radiol 11: 21–25
12. Andersson R, Janzon M, Sundberg I, Bengmark S (1989) Management of pancreatic pseudocysts. Br J Surg 76: 550–552
13. Altimari A, Aranha GV, Greenlee HB, Prinz RA (1986) Results of cystoduodenostomy for treatment of pancreatic pseudocysts. Am Surg 52: 438–441
14. Campion JP, Bardaxoglou E, Caillon P, Faroux R, Bourdonnec P (1989) Surgical treatment of chronic pancreatitis. Indications and results. An experience of 246 cases. Chirurgie 115: 123–131

Tumor Therapy by Ethanol Injection: Results and Indications

T. Livraghi

Percutaneous ethanol injection (PEI) is an inexpensive and easy therapeutic technique performed under ultrasound guidance. Ultrasound real-time control permits recognition of the target, correct centering of the fine needle in the preselected area, and evaluation of the appropriate quantity of ethanol to inject. The toxic effects of ethanol injected into neoplastic lesions have been assessed in animals and on operative specimens from humans. Alcohol enters the cells by diffusion and produces immediate coagulation necrosis followed by the formation of granulation tissue and fibrosis and by partial or complete thrombosis of small vessels. The phenomena are the outcome of cellular dehydration and protein denaturation. Primary and metastatic neoplasms of the liver are the pathologies treated by PEI.

The rationale for treatment of small hepatic cell carcinoma (HCC) in cirrhosis rests on the following points:

1) initially the expansive form of HCC shows regional growth;
2) ultrasound screening of a cirrhosis population permits one to recognize HCC at its initial stage;
3) ethanol shows a selective diffusion in HCC because of its softer consistency;
4) PEI does not involve loss of cirrhotic tissue as does surgery, and thus liver failure is not hastened;
5) PEI does not present serious complications in comparison with perioperative morbidity and mortality;
6) a high rate (55 % – 70 %) of livers treated with any kind of therapy produces other lesions in 2–3 years.

Four differing 3-year survival rates (Kaplan-Meier method) in patients with single or multiple HCC under 5 cm are available: 65 % was reported by Ebara in 95 patients (single plus multiple, under 3 cm), 58 % by Livraghi in 70 patients (72 % in single and 25 % in multiple), 68 % by Shiina in 50 patients (68 % in single and 37 % in multiple and 60 % by an Italian multicenter study in 178 patients (70 % in single and 27 % in multiple). The survival rate in 27 comparable, untreated patients reported by Ebara was 7 %. The survival rate for a total of 517 comparable patients treated by surgery ranged from 41 % to 76 %. In conclusion, the survival of patients treated by PEI or by surgery was similar (overall average: 68 % and 56 %, respectively).

In our opinion, the indications for PEI are:

1) inoperable single HCC under 5–6 cm;
2) operable single HCC under 5 cm presenting the same adverse prognostic factor for resection (difficult surgical approach, important loss of cirrhotic tissue, no capsule, old age, Child's B class);
3) multiple HCC, in which any method is merely palliative, in association with intraarterial therapies;
4) adenomatous hyperplastic nodules, confirmed as precursor of HCC (in this pathology surgical treatment is a problem because resection of a precancerous lesion is considered inadvisable in patients with high surgical risk).

The rationale for the treatment of metastatic lesions is strictly limited by the natural course of the disease because PEI is a local therapy. A study carried out on 14 patients with lesions of differing origins was reported in our series: a complete response was obtained in 11 (9 less than 2 cm) out of 21 lesions, with a maximum recurrence-free follow-up of 40 months in metastasis of gastrinoma. The pathologic baseline values of CEA were lowered in all patients but one and in one case normalized for periods ranging from 2 to 6 months. Subsequent elevations were attributed to regrowth of the treated lesion, recurrence of the primary, extrahepatic metastases, or new liver metastases. It is difficult or impossible to establish whether, how much, and in which cases patient survival was lengthened. Arguably, the same prognostic factors that are applied in the selection of candidates for surgical resection played a fundamental role in these cases too. On the strength of the results obtained in patients with synchronous, even unifocal, or metachronous multifocal lesions there do not seem to be real indications for PEI or for the mounting of controlled trials, quite apart from the cost and the difficulty of finding truly comparable patients. In practice, however, it was hard to deny treatment to patients, for example, with two small inoperable metachronous lesions. On the other hand, in patients with a single metachronous lesion of less than 4 cm that is inoperable or where surgery is refused, PEI might find a place among the therapeutic options for which a controlled trial might be set up. All the endocrine metastases presented a complete remission. This was because of their small size, their slow growth, and probably their hypervascularity. Thus in endocrine metastases PEI may also find a use, possibly in association with the nonsurgical therapies that have long been in use. In conclusion, data obtained were relevant to a continuance of PEI application on a very targeted basis, possibly with a control arm.

PEI is a safe procedure as no important complications occurred in more than 1000 sessions.

Intravascular Scanning Devices and Their Clinical Value

K. Bom, C. T. Lancée, W. J. Gussenhoven, J. Roelandt, W. Li, and M. G. M. de Kroon

Reports of intraluminal diagnostic ultrasound methods date back to the early 1950s. In those days researchers described echographic methods with the acoustic element mounted either on a catheter tip, gastroscope pipe, or other means for intraluminal diagnostic applications of ultrasound. One of the compelling reasons for intraluminal approach at that time was the low sensitivity of the available echo transducers and therefore the need to closely approach the organs to be studied. With the success of noninvasive ultrasound diagnostic methods very little was heard about the invasive methods over recent decades. However, with the introduction of interventional vascular methods this changed about 5 years ago. For instance, with lumen dilatation, the initial success rate has been encouraging. However, approximately one-third of the treated lesions show signs of restenosis within a certain period. Other recently developed therapeutic methods also show a restenosis rate which is approximately in this order. The optimal use of these devices for any specific obstruction is not well understood. More knowledge of morphology and geometry of the obstruction is of paramount importance to understand new interventional methods.

Since ultrasound allows observation of cross-sectional information, it was logical that renewed efforts on the use of catheter tip based instruments would be spent. The principal clinical problem in developing intra-arterial imaging techniques has been the miniaturization of the accoustic components inside the catheter.

Intravascular imaging systems are based on earlier described methods and consist of three types. The first is a rotating tip system in which a very flexible shaft contains the electric wire for the transducer, and the transducer rotates together with this shaft. Usually the tip is covered with an acoustically transparent dome which allows the beam to pass without causing reverberation echoes. The angle between the sound beam and the dome is slightly off perpendicular to avoid reverberation of echoes from the dome wall. Instead of the transducer element itself, the second combines a fixed stationary acoustic element with a rotating mirror. Both systems must be filled with an acoustic coupling liquid which is injected just prior to the clinical procedure. Air bubbles may cause malfunction of the system, and in this case a short additional flush of saline may solve the problem.

Since the catheter must follow a tortuous path, as a result the beam deflection on the display may not correspond with the acoustic beam deflection and thus can create minor image artifacts. In both mechanically driven catheter tip systems a very flexible drive shaft is used. Rotational power from a proximally mounted motor is transferred via this shaft to the rotating echo tip or mirror. To visualize curved arteries such as the coronary arteries a compromise is necessary between the required low flexural rigidity and the high torsional rigidity. Shaft situations can be simulated with phantom images showing artifacts from a catheter in a straight line or a catheter inserted in the glass model of an aorta and coronary artery mimicking the same tortuous path as in the clinical situation. An illustration with a test object containing eight wires equally distributed over 360° is presented in Fig. 1. The artifacts for a flexible drive shaft are shown under three conditions.

The third intravascular technique is based on electronically switched phased arrays. A number of elements are mounted cylindrically on the outer boundary of the catheter. This construction is similar to that described in 1972 by Bom [1], who initiated a program to develop two-dimensional real-time invasive ultrasound using a 32-element phased array transducer with a diameter of 3.2 mm mounted at the tip of a 9-F catheter. The array was designed to use subgroups of elements with phased delay – in a rapid manner. This early system used analog delay lines and switches outside the catheter. This allowed a frame rate of 196 frames per second. In today's systems internal switching devices minimize the number of wires inside the catheter. The delay is introduced subsequently in the image reconstruction algorithm. The advantages of these electronic devices are that a central guidewire can be easily allowed, and that no moving parts exist.

As in all echo systems a short transmission of acoustic energy takes place during pulse transmission. This causes a transient effect or amplifier

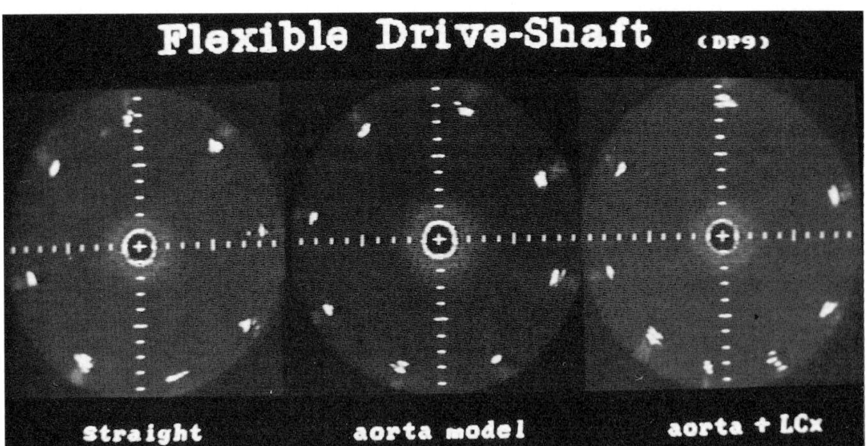

Fig. 1. Phantom images obtained from a test object. From left to right: the catheter in a straight line, the catheter in a glass model of the aorta, and the catheter in a glass model of aorta plus coronary artery

saturation during which no echoes can be received. Only after this transient effect does the acoustic element start its role as receiver. The principle is illustrated in Fig. 2. As can be seen the mirror type has the shortest dead zone, completely inside the catheter. The electronic system with the multiplicity of elements positioned at the outer circumference produces an "acoustic diameter" which is slightly larger than the catheter itself.

As a further comparison it should be mentioned that the electronically switched catheter systems incorporate possibilities for variable focusing of the acoustic beam. On the other hand, the acoustic beam is a three-dimensional definition. The mechanical systems usually operate with a small disclike acoustic element which allows an optimal acoustic beam in all cross-sectional axial planes through the sound beam. From this it can be concluded that image quality for proximal structures in mechanically rotated systems is better than the image quality obtained in the same situation with a phased array device.

Excellent correlation of histologic and echographic images as obtained in vitro at 40 MHz has been described by Gussenhoven et al. [2]. It appeared that, based on the typical histologic differences found in the composition of the media, accurate distinction was possible between the different types of arteries studies. The wall of muscular arteries presented as a typical three-layered structure. The elastic artery, conversely, was recognized by absence of the typical hypoechoic media. The presence of elastin fibers in the media of an elastic artery resulted in a significant amount of acoustic backscatter, the power level of which was comparable to that of the surrounding tissue. Echographically speaking, therefore, the media could not

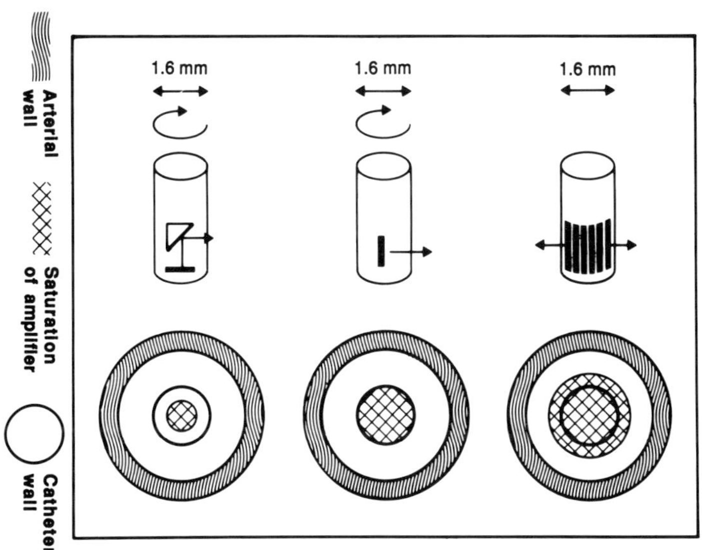

Fig. 2. The transient effect or acoustic "dead zone" as present in various systems

be distinguished in elastic arteries. Plaque could be distinguished as follows:

1) absence of echoes is seen in significant deposit of lipids,
2) diffuse intimal thickening yields soft echoes,
3) collagen-rich fibrous tissue yields bright echoes, and
4) calcium causes bright echoes with shadowing behind the lesion.

Besides the observed differences in acoustic response of morphologically different tissues, significant variations in backscatter power are found in both media and internal elastic lamina due to variations in the angle of incidence. This angle dependence is caused by the dominant orientation of fibers in tissue layers and by the shape and size of various scattering particles. Results indicate that long microscopic structures with one main orientation are responsible for the backscattered signal, and that the angle-dependent response is related to the histologically determined orientation of these fibers [3]. An example of the normalized power versus angle curve of the muscular media is presented Fig. 3. The results are shown from a variation of angles of incidence in the long axis or axial plane and a variation of the angle of incidence in a plane perpendicular to the long axis of the artery, the tangential plane.

Another area of interest is the quantification of intravascular ultrasonic images. Quantitative assessment of lumen area, lesion area, and area obstruction can be performed by tracing the boundaries of the free lumen and original lumen. In both in vitro and in vivo studies, quantitative assessment of intravascular ultrasound agreed well with histology and angiography, except for the 17% underestimate in histologic lumen area measurements. The

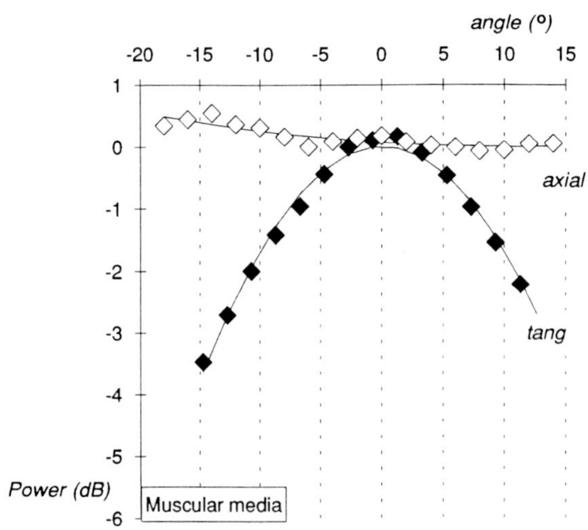

Fig. 3. The normalized ultrasonic backscatter power versus angle shown for the muscular media, resulting in two perpendicular planes (see text)

underestimate by histology can probably be attributed to the fixation and tissue processing during histologic preparation of the specimen. After this procedure the shape of the vessel lumen may alter due to tissue shrinkage. For comparison to angiography it should be noted that intravascular ultrasound is a tomographic technique and angiography a shadow technique. Thus, identical results may be expected only in vessels with a circular geometry. The investigated accuracy and reproducibility of intravascular images has been described by Li [4].

In many research centers today intravascular echography is being used to improve understanding of the interventional procedure. Image quality is improving rapidly, and with this the possibilities for determining more accurately the situation before and after the therapeutic intervention procedure. An example of this is given in Fig. 4, where the luminal area has changed following balloon angioplasty. Figure 5 illustrates that the increase in free luminal area can be quantified by analyzing echograms acquired before and after intervention from the same arterial position as described above.

These and similar studies will teach the users of intravascular echography about the interventional technique. Of course we are only at the beginning of

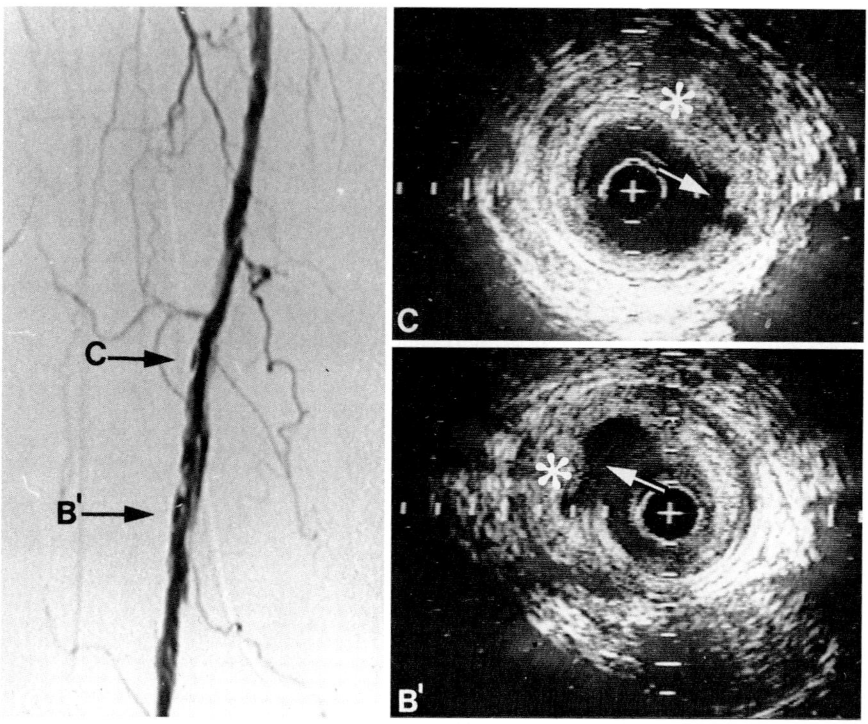

Fig. 4. Example of two positions in the femoral artery as imaged after balloon dilatation. Notice the apparent rupture *(arrow)*

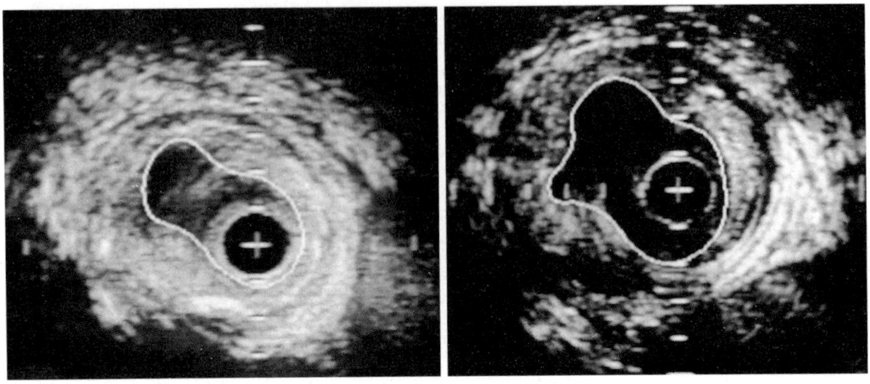

Fig. 5. Example of quantification by contour analysis. *Left,* before intervention (free lumen area 10.6 mm^2); *right,* after intervention (free lumen area 16.6 mm^2). The area of free lumen was increased by 57 % as a result of the intervention

the clinical use of intravascular ultrasound, which shows much promise. However, it will take time before the enormous potential of these new methods is appreciated, and the optimal clinical use becomes clear.

Acknowledgement. These investigations were supported by a grant from the Netherlands Technology Foundation (STW, grant RGN79.1257).

References

1. Bom N, Lancée CT, Van Egmond FC (1972) An ultrasonic intracardiac scanner. Ultrasonics 10: 72–76
2. Gussenhoven WJ, Essed CE, Frietman P, Mastik F, Lancée CT, Slager CJ, Serruys PW, Gerritsen P, Pieterman H, Bom N (1989) Intravascular echographic assessment of vessel wall characteristics: a correlation with histology. Int J Card Imaging 4: 105–116
3. De Kroon MGM, Van der Wal LF, Gussenhoven WJ, Rijsterborgh H, Bom N (1991) Backscatter directivity and integrated backscatter power of arterial tissue. In: Bom N, Roelandt J, Gussenhoven WJ (eds) Intravascular ultrasound. Kluwer, Dordrecht, pp 265–275
4. Li W, Gussenhoven WJ, Bosch JG, Mastik F, Reiber JHC, Bom N (1991) A computer-aided analysis system for the quantitative assessment of intravascular ultrasound images. In: Computers in cardiology 1990. IEEE Computer Society Press, Los Alamitos, pp 333–336

Advances in Ultrasound: Contrast Agents and Endoluminal Ultrasound

B. B. Goldberg and J.-B. Liu

Endoluminal Ultrasound

The concept of placing transducers within various lumina of the body goes back to the actual beginnings of ultrasound in the late 1940s and early 1950s. Wild, in the United States at that time, developed a small transducer which he placed in the rectum to evaluate the mucosa of the bowel in an attempt to identify early cancer [60]. Since that time other pioneers have developed miniaturized transducers, including von Micsky in the United States who developed a rigid ultrasound probe that was inserted into the endometrial canal [58]. Holm in Denmark developed a rigid miniaturized transducer which could be inserted through the urethra into the urinary bladder to evaluate and stage urinary bladder cancer [27]. These early attempts were limited by the technology available at the time. The possibility of miniaturizing transducers to the point that they could be placed within blood vessels was first conceived by Bom in Holland in the 1970s [3]. At that time, he developed a transducer about 2 mm in diameter which could be advanced through a blood vessel into the heart. Since that time a number of researchers and companies have been working on further perfecting this approach. It was not until the past several years that miniature ultrasound transducers contained within catheters became commercially available. The motive behind these developments by a number of companies, both small and large, was the perceived need to find a way to better evaluate the extent of thrombus within arteries. Over the past several years there have been a number of papers, in the United States and abroad, reporting results of studies in both animals and humans pertaining to the usefulness of these flexible transducer-containing catheters. Initial reports have shown great promise for being able to not only diagnose but also to determine the extent of thrombus in a variety of vessels in the body. This approach shows promise in being able to monitor the removal of plaque (atherectomy) and the dilatation of areas of stenosis (angioplasty) [28, 34, 39, 45, 61].

With the development of any new ultrasound instrument or transducer there is the possibility of utilizing it in a different way from that originally planned. This is what occurred in our facility during the past 2 years. Working together with a variety of physicians, both radiologists and nonradiologists, a series of protocols were developed to evaluate the potential nonvascular uses of these new miniature transducers housed within flexible catheters. It should be pointed out that the concept of placing transducers within lumina has already been established through the use of ultrasound transducers incorporated into flexible gastroscopes. Although not popular in the United States, these transducer-containing gastroscopes have been used extensively in Japan and Europe over the past decade. They can be inserted through the esophagus, into the stomach, and even into the duodenum to produce cross-sectional ultrasound images not only of the walls of the esophagus and stomach but also beyond [16, 25, 41]. This approach has proven useful in identifing submucosal masses and differentiating the cause of extrinsic mass effect on these structures, such as enlarged lymph nodes and vessels. In addition, when malignancy is present, this technique has proven useful in determining tumor extension as well as the involvement of adjacent lymph nodes [5]. Abnormalities in adjacent organs, such as the pancreas, have also been evaluated with this method [50]. Thus, there was already a basis upon which to predict the success of utilizing the much smaller transducer-containing catheters in various regions of the body.

While there are several endoluminal ultrasound instruments as well as a variety of catheters available, for our research we have used the Diasonics IVUS (Milpitas, CA) in association with Medi-tech/Boston Scientific (Watertown, MA). This equipment uses a single-element transducer that revolves at more than 30 frames per second, producing a real-time cross-sectional image offset at 10° from perpendicular. A variety of catheters are available, with new ones planned for the future, including those of 4.8, 6, and 9 F and containing either a 20- or a 12.5-MHz transducer. They are either blunt tipped or over guide wires which are useful in advancing into smaller lumina (Fig. 1). As with any new technology, animal research was initially carried out to test not only the feasibility but also the safety. In our initial research [22] we demonstrated the feasibility of using these catheters in a variety of nonvascular regions of the body. In the initial set of experiments 6-F

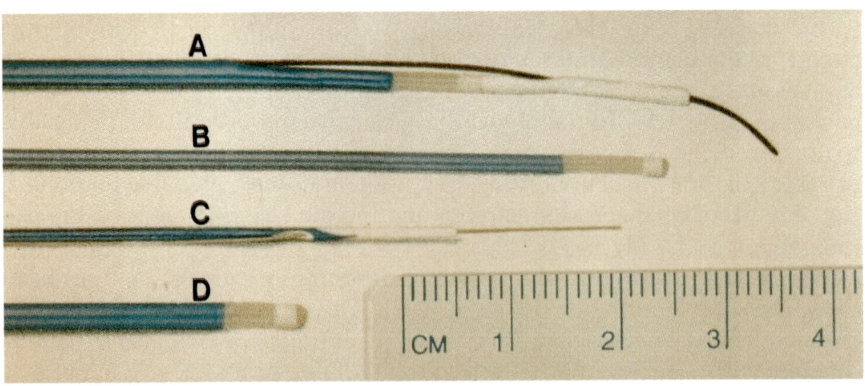

Fig. 1. Variety of transducer-containing catheters: *A*, 6-F over a guidewire; *B*, 6-F blunt tip; *C*, 4.8-F over a guidewire; *D*, 9-F blunt tip

catheters and 20-MHz transducers were utilized. Later, we worked successfully with 9-F catheters and 12.5-MHz transducers. In the initial animal experiments it was possible to pass these catheters into the urethra, urinary bladder, ureter, and renal pelvis as well as the endometrial canal and fallopian tube. In addition, using a surgical approach it was possible to pass these transducer-containing catheters into the biliary and pancreatic ducts. These transducers produced 360° cross-sectional ultrasound images perpendicular to the long axis of the catheter. It was possible to record not only reflections from the walls of the lumina in which they were inserted but also beyond these structures, including visualization of adjacent lymph nodes, muscles, and blood vessels [22].

Upon completion of our animal experiments we concluded that this approach could readily be used in humans. No damage was produced by the catheters and none would be expected since they are smooth-walled and have been used for a variety of intravascular procedures. The catheters are, of course, sterilized and in the case of humans not reused. As with the animal experiments, the University Research Committee approved our various protocols, including the consent forms which allowed us to proceed. During the past 2 years, a wide variety of catheter insertions have been performed throughout the body in over 100 patients.

Urological Uses

This has been our most successful area of evaluation to date with some established uses and others showing significant promise [20]. These catheters are no more than 2–3 mm in diameter and can be easily passed into the urethra without the need for dilatation. In the urethra it has been possible to visualize various anatomical structures and to delineate areas of abnormality, including plaque or fibrosis. In addition, as it passes through the prostatic portion of the urethra, this structure can be imaged, especially the periurethral portion. The uniformity and nonuniformity of the prostate gland in this region has been clearly identified. It should be pointed out that the posterior and lateral aspects are best delineated with transrectal ultrasound. However, initial results suggest that the more central portion may well be best evaluated with the endourethral approach. It could also be used before, during, and after transurethral prostatectomy. In one case it was possible to monitor the extent of tissue removal.

In the urinary bladder it is possible to visualize tumors and to evaluate the extent of their invasiveness (Fig. 2). It should also be possible not only to aid in the staging of bladder tumors in terms of their penetration into and beyond the bladder wall but also to image adjacent lymph nodes. It should be pointed out that rigid endourethral transducers have been utilized in the past, but with these small flexible catheters it is a much easier procedure to perform since there is no need for urethral dilatation.

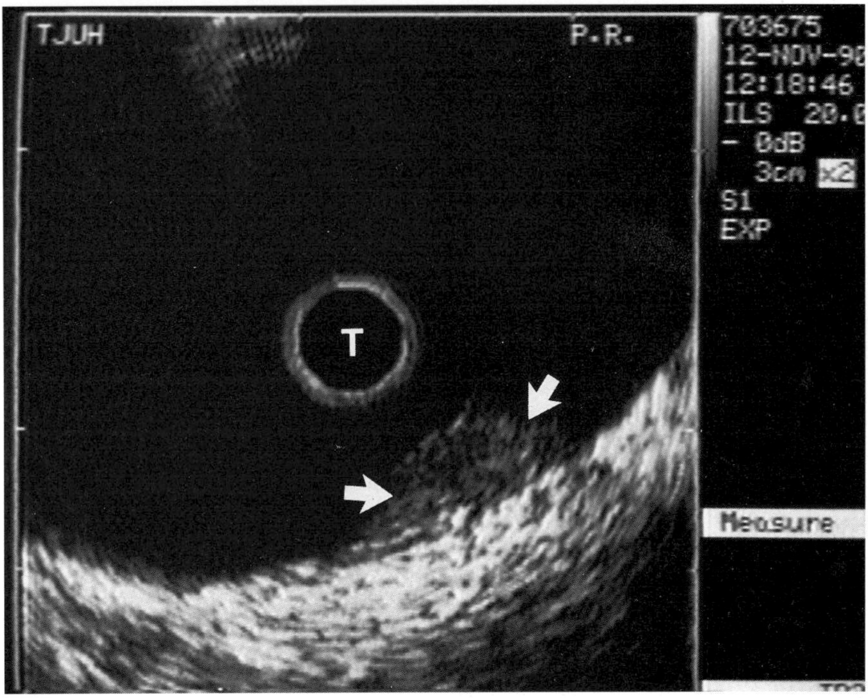

Fig. 2. Urinary bladder tumor *(arrows)* is seen arising from the posterior wall with no evidence of invasion. *T,* transducer

In evaluating the ureter it is important to work along with the urologist, who must first position a cystoscope. These small transducer-containing catheters can then be easily inserted through the cystoscope and directed through the ureteral orifice into the ureter (Fig. 3). In general, this procedure is accomplished in only a few minutes. Once within the ureter, it is possible to detect and differentiate a wide variety of abnormalities. It is in the evaluation of the ureter that this method has already established its importance in our institution. For instance, with this method it is possible to detect stones embedded within the mucosa of the ureter and renal pelvis (Fig. 4). Prior to this method, direct endoscopic approaches could only visualize the surface of the mucosa of the ureter and renal pelvis.

With this approach it has been possible to visualize abnormalities beyond the ureter, including crossing vessels and enlarged lymph nodes (Fig. 5). In fact, our urologist no longer makes an incision into the mucosa to relieve obstruction due to extrinsic vessel or mass unless endoluminal ultrasound is performed. For instance, if there is a crossing vessel the urologist takes additional care when incising the mucosa, which is only a few millimeters in thickness, avoiding the possibility of entering the adjacent vessel. This approach has also been able to identify the presence and extent of ureteral tumors (Fig. 6). Endoluminal ultrasound appears to add information not

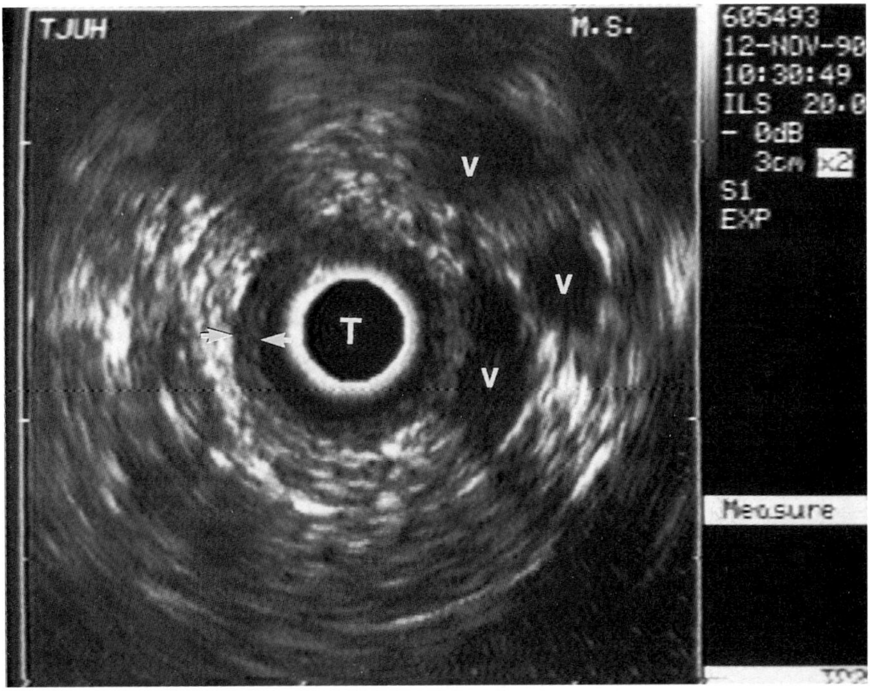

Fig. 3. Endoluminal transducer-containing catheter *(T)* positioned within the ureter delineates several adjacent blood vessels *(V)*. Note the normal ureteral wall *(arrows)* and the minimal amount of urine *(echo-free region)* adjacent to the transducer

available with the other imaging techniques such as standard ultrasound, computed tomography, magnetic resonance imaging, and retrograde urography. Even ureteroscopy cannot provide this information since it can only visualize abnormalities that involve the mucosa surface.

From our initial results we can already predict that nonvascular endoluminal ultrasound will become an important part of the urologic examination. It is important for those performing ultrasound, i.e., radiologists, to realize this and to act accordingly.

Gynecological Uses

These miniature transducer-containing catheters have been passed through the cervical os without the need for dilatation, unless there is a stricture present. It has been possible to image the endometrium and adjacent myometrium. Initial results have shown it to be useful in helping to differentiate many causes of uterine bleeding [23]. Endoluminal ultrasound images have demonstrated submucosal myomas, endometrial polyps, and synechia as well as endometrial and cervical carcinoma. In addition, in the

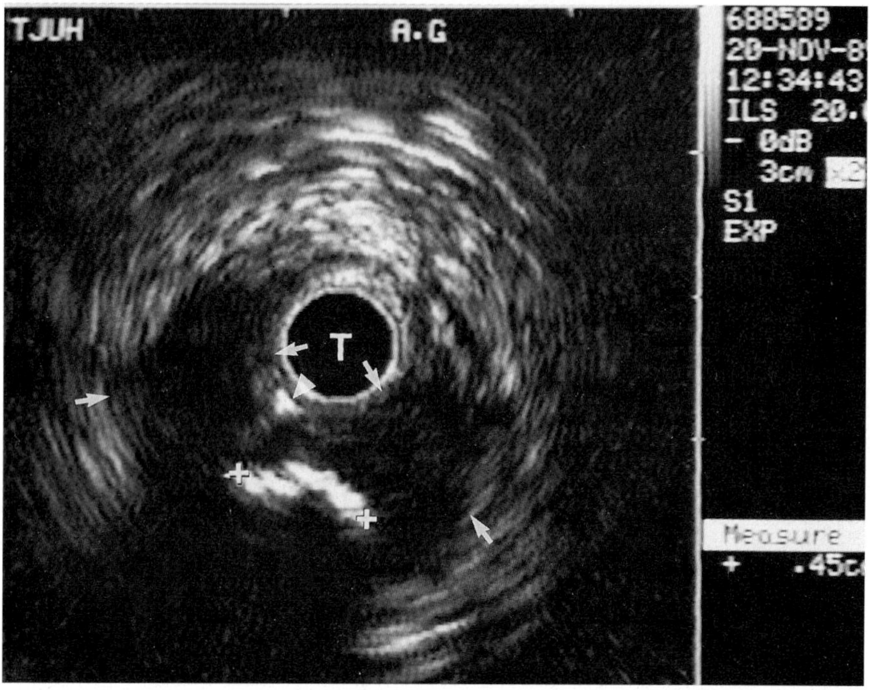

Fig. 4. Endoluminal ultrasound transducer *(T)* within the ureter demonstrates hypoechoic edematous mucosa *(arrows)* in which is embedded a stone *(crosses)*, producing distal acoustic shadowing. The bright reflection *(arrowhead)* adjacent to the transducer is produced by a guidewire. (From [20] with permission)

cervical region Nabothian cysts have been clearly identified. This technique was performed in a number of cases both prior to and following surgery. Subsequent cross-sectional anatomical slices allow us to correlate the ultrasound findings with the pathology results. Close correlation of those results confirmed our ability to delineate a variety of abnormalities. For instance, with myomas a typical hypoechoic appearance was seen. Their relationship adjacent to the endometrium could also be clearly identified. A hyperechoic polyp, as well as synechia, could also be imaged. It was possible to demonstrate the presence of both endometrial and cervical cancer (Fig. 7).

While still more cases need to be performed to confirm the usefulness of this approach relative to endovaginal ultrasound, our initial results are most promising. The concept is that of being able to use a higher frequency than is used with endovaginal ultrasound, i.e., 12.5 and 20 MHz, allowing us to image smaller abnormalities.

Preliminary work has been carried out utilizing these transducer-containing catheters in the evaluation of the fallopian tube. The catheter is directed

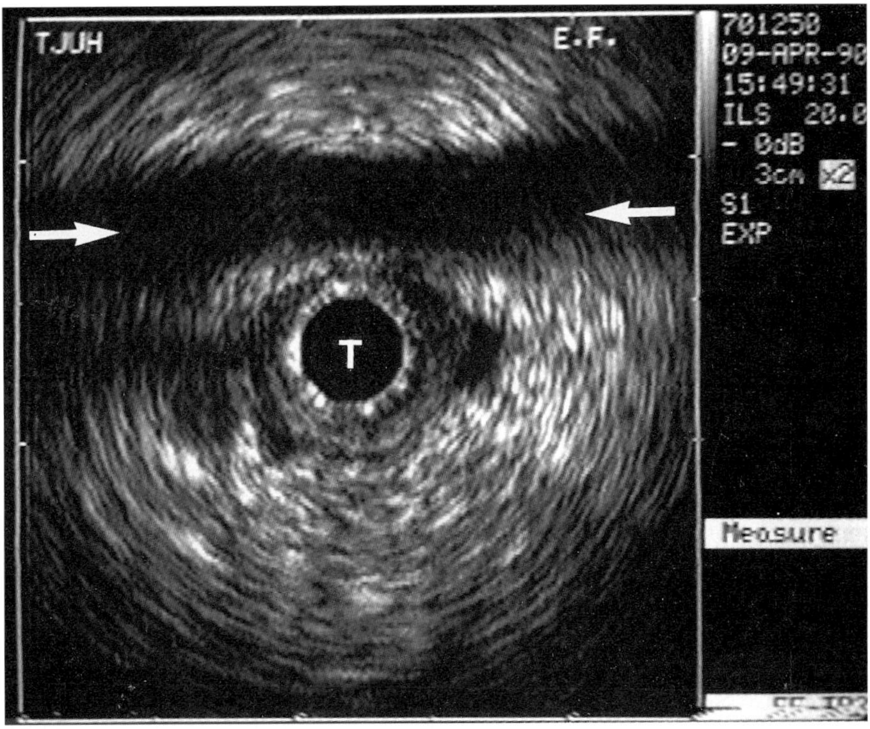

Fig. 5. A tubular echogenic structure *(arrows)* is seen just adjacent to the proximal ureter, consistent with a crossing vessel, which was the cause of the patient's hydronephrosis. *T*, transducer. (From [20] with permission)

through a hysteroscope into the fallopian tube. With this approach it may be possible to detect infertility. External approaches, with insertion of these catheters through a laparoscope, are also under investigation. These approaches could prove helpful in the detection of small ovarian or tubal abnormalities, including early ectopic pregnancies. Initial work has already been carried out by inserting these catheters into the endometrial canal to image earlier gestation just prior to abortion.

Gastrointestinal Uses

As has been described previously, the concept of using endoluminal ultrasound within the GI tract has already shown feasibility with transducers attached to gastroscopes. In cooperation with our interventional imaging physicians, we have been able to pass the flexible transducer-containing catheters through previously established tubes in the biliary system to demonstrate the presence and extent of cholangiocarcinoma, including the

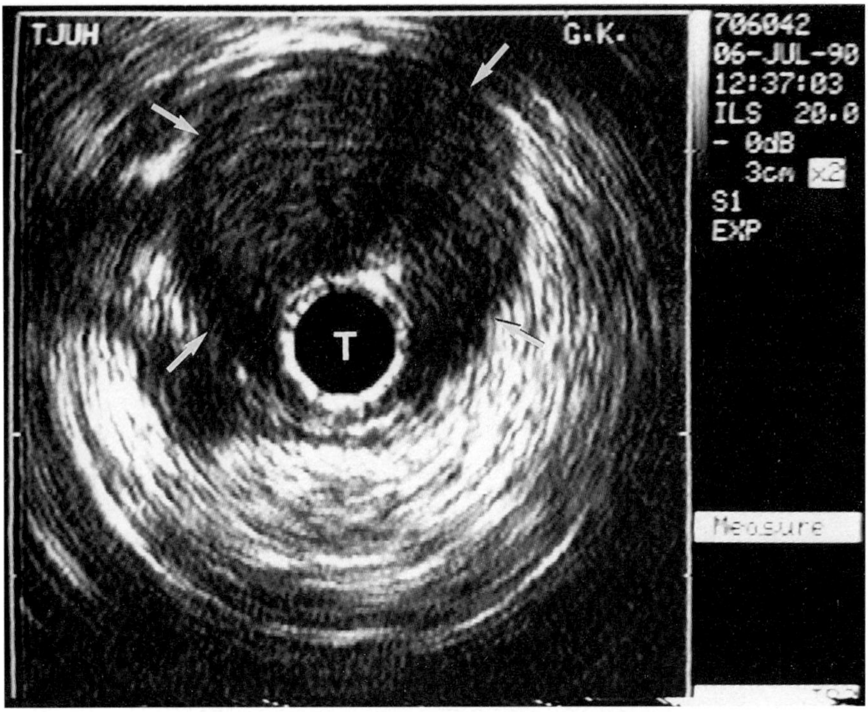

Fig. 6. The transducer-containing catheter *(T)* demonstrates a solid mass *(arrows)* arising from a portion of the ureteral wall, consistent with a diagnosis of ureteral tumor, which was confirmed by subsequent biopsy

visualization of adjacent lymph nodes and vessels. Working with surgeons in the operating room we have passed these catheters into the pancreatic duct and demonstrated the presence of tumors and stones. They have also been passed into the adjacent small bowel, with clear delineation of the various layers of the wall of the small bowel. These catheters can also be passed with relative ease into the esophagus. Due to the relatively high ultrasound frequencies utilized it is possible to image five layers; that is, the hyperechogenic mucosa (including submucosa) and adventitia as well as two hypoechogenic muscle layers (circular and longitudinal) separated by a thin echogenic intermuscular connective tissue layer (Fig. 8). Standard esophageal endosonography using transducers housed in flexible gastroscopes have not been able to show this detail, most likely due to the lower frequencies utilized. With these smaller, higher frequency transducers it was possible to demonstrate and diagnose a variety of abnormalities, including esophageal carcinoma, achalasia, and scleroderma (Fig. 9). Mucosal and submucosal thickening due to inflammation was also imaged, including the detection of dilated vessels in the submucosa.

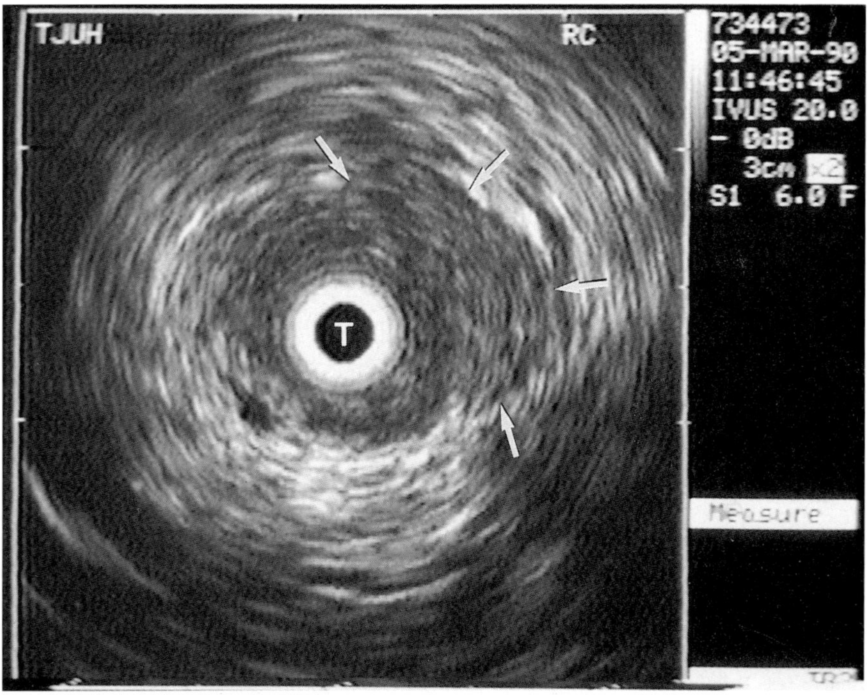

Fig. 7. Endoluminal transducer-containing catheter *(T)* located within the endometrial canal demonstrates the presence of irregular solid mass *(arrows)* extending from the endometrium into the myometrium. This was confirmed pathologically to be a grade 1 endometrial carcinoma with invasion of the adjacent one-third of the myometrium. (From [23] with permission)

It is envisioned that it will eventually be possible to pass these catheters through openings in a gastroscope and, as is done with ERCP, to place them in the biliary or pancreatic ducts. This approach should provide more information than is now available since it can visualize beyond the wall of the lumen. In the future it may also be possible to have a long enough catheter to be fed through the entire small bowel, evaluating for a variety of intestinal abnormalities.

Other Potential Uses

It was possible to advance these catheters into such regions as the mediastinum and abdomen. Our initial work has shown that they can be passed through a mediastinoscope. This approach has allowed the surgeon to more easily detect the exact position of lymph nodes prior to their biopsy. The position of the blood vessels, as well as other vital structures and their relationship to areas of abnormality, is easily determined. This technique

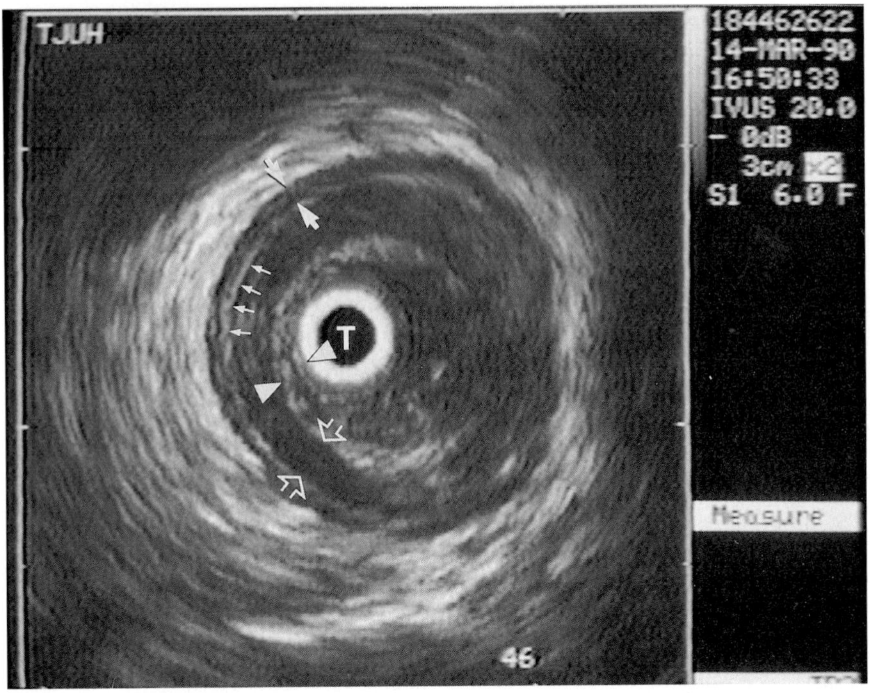

Fig. 8. The transducer-containing catheter *(T)* positioned within the distal esophagus delineates the various normal layers, including the two hypoechogenic circular muscular *(open arrows)* and longitudinal muscular *(large arrows)* layers separated by a thin echogenic intermuscular connective tissue layer *(small arrows)*. The relative hyperechogenic mucosal and adjacent submucosal layers *(arrowheads)* as well as the hyperechogenic adventitia are also clearly seen

shows promise in decreasing the length of time spent by the surgeon in identifying and biopsying lymph nodes and mediastinal masses. These catheters have also been placed within the surgically exposed spinal canal. In these cases it is possible to image the spinal cord. This approach should prove useful in the detection of bone fragments and a variety of cord abnormalities.

This same approach shows promise as an aid during laparoscopy for evaluating a variety of pelvic and abdominal organs. Protocols are underway for working with a variety of surgeons and gynecologists to evaluate this approach. The concept of placing these transducer-containing catheters in areas of suspected abnormalities should provide additional information, not available using standard laparoscopic techniques, by providing ultrasound images of structures beneath the surface of the region of concern. Placement of these catheters into abscesses or other types of collections that are being drained could prove useful in determining the extent of the cavity and changes in response to treatment.

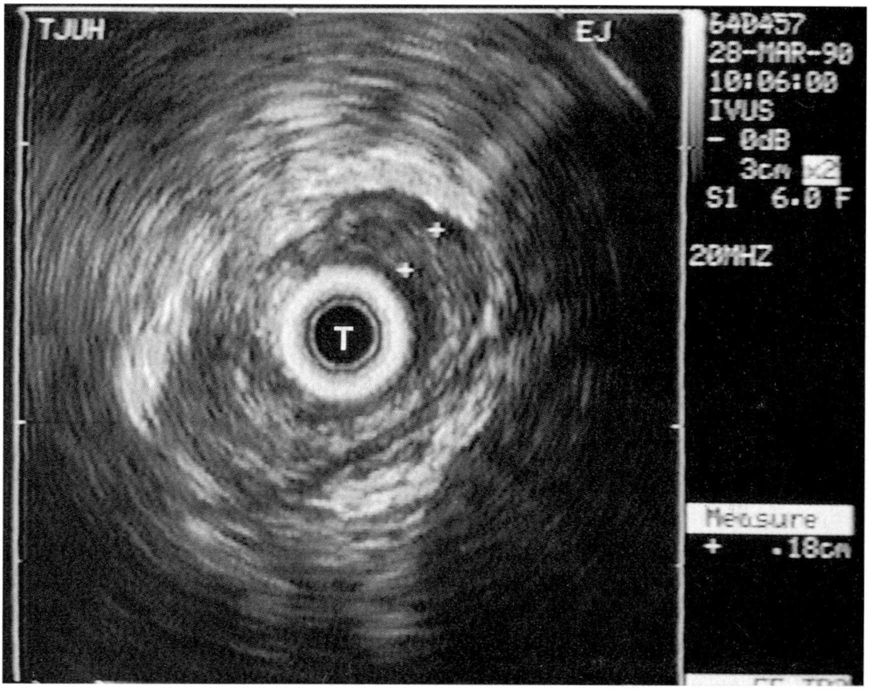

Fig. 9. Endoluminal transducer-containing catheter *(T)* located in the distal esophagus in a patient with scleroderma demonstrates diffusely increased echogenicity of the esophageal wall *(crosses)*. The normal delineation of the various wall structures have disappeared

Summary

In conclusion, these specially developed transducer-containing catheters, intended originally for placement in blood vessels, show great promise as important new tools in a wide variety of nonvascular lumina and surgically created openings in many areas of the body. What originated as an idea to look into the potential nonvascular uses through initial animal experiments has led to our development of 15 different protocols, many of which have been reviewed here.

Ultrasound Contrast Agents

The concept of ultrasound contrast agents was first introduced through the work of Gramiak in 1968 [24]. In patients with normal aortic valves who were undergoing ascending aortography, saline was injected into the supravalvular region during continuous M-mode echocardiographic recording. The injected saline was detected as a cloud of echoes contained within the lumen of the aortic root. At that time, Gramiak speculated that the saline-produced echoes were arising from microbubbles of gas. Subsequent reports substantiated that the reflectivity was due to the presence of microbubbles of gas which went back into solution over time [13, 62]. Other investigators subsequently used such solutions as indocine green to confirm the presence of such cardiac abnormalities as shunts and valvular insufficiency [11, 32]. Noncardiac uses for ultrasound contrast agents have also been reported [18, 19]. Since then, various other solutions have proven to be potentially useful as ultrasound contrast agents by virtue of their ability to trap gas microbubbles. In fact, almost any solution which is agitated and then injected into a vein or artery produces echoes. The intensity of the echoes varies with the type of solution utilized, with the most viscous solutions containing the most microbubbles.

Over the years, sonification of solutions, including dextrose, sorbitol, and renographin, has become the most common approach to the generation of ultrasound contrast agents [29]. Most of the early work with these agents was done to evaluate a variety of cardiographic abnormalities. Gramiak used them aid in identifying the pulmonic valve. Others have used them to evaluate valvular regurgitation and to confirm the presence as well as the size of shunts at both the atrial and ventricular levels [48, 51]. This initial research recorded the actual increase in reflectivity from within the cavities. Recently, the same concept has been used with Doppler to increase its signal strength [1]. This approach has helped to more clearly demonstrate cardiac shunts as well as flow reversal and in one report, to increase the ability to detect coronary artery blood flow [33, 56]. One of the problems with these solutions that use gas bubbles formed principally via agitation is that the bubbles vary in size and are often too large to pass through the pulmonary capillaries. However, this approach is still being used. For instance, bubbles of gas have been injected directly into vessels to enhance the reflectivity of the structures they perfuse. This approach has been used intraoperatively to better detect small hepatic carcinomas [54]. Carbon dioxide is mixed with physiologic saline and injected through a catheter placed in the hepatic artery. Real-time ultrasound monitoring of the liver showed an immediate increase in echogenicity of the liver parenchyma which, after a few minutes, decreased at a faster rate than the tumor, allowing for its better visualization. Although there has been concern about the possibility of these bubbles occluding capillaries in the brain or other organs, several reports have concluded that these agents are relatively safe [4, 17]. More importantly, injections of these types of ultrasound contrast agents can occur only near the region of interest since the microbubbles tend to go back into solution after a relatively short distance.

Researchers have continued to seek other methods of producing and maintaining, over longer distances, uniform small bubble sizes capable of passing through the capillary system [12, 49]. The most promising work in this area has consisted of microbubbles of gas incorporated within either a sugar matrix or human albumin [2, 30, 53]. Not only can these agents last for a much longer time, but their more uniform smaller size allows them to pass through the capillaries. They remain intact long enough to be able to circulate at least once through the circulatory system. In addition to ongoing research in the development of improved microbubble-containing ultrasound contrast agents, researchers have looked into other approaches, including the use of collagen spheres as well as solutions of various osmolarity [8, 42, 43, 57]. In addition, perflourochemicals have also been utilized as ultrasound contrast agents [37].

Two approaches have been followed: (a) in a fashion similar to X-ray arteriography, increasing the reflectivity of the blood, and (b) enhancing the Doppler signals [44, 45]. It is non-organ-specific. The other type is organ- or tumor-specific since it tends to collect within or around abnormalities within such structures as the liver and spleen, increasing the difference in reflectivity (echogenicity) between the normal and adjacent abnormal tissue [35].

A variety of approaches have been used, including the use of aqueous solutions, emulsions, suspensions, and encapsulated bubbles. Initial work in the area of aqueous solutions was carried out by Ophir, who demonstrated that there was an increase in echogenicity within the kidneys, both in vitro and in vivo, when they were intravascularly injected [43]. A variety of solutions were tried, including sodium citrate and calcium disodium EDTA. However, the amount of solution needed to produce significant enhancement as well as concern over the toxicity of some of these solutions has limited the usefulness of this approach [44]. Fink used emulsions of lipid in the hope that it would have the same effect as fatty infiltration of the liver by increasing echogenicity of the tissue [14]. It was found that the amount of lipid emulsion required to be injected to mimic fatty infiltration of the liver would be prohibitively high.

The use of colloidal suspensions has shown some success in increasing the backscatter (echogenicity) of the tissue as well as enhancing the Doppler signal. Initial work by Ophir showed enhancement in canine livers in vivo using collagen microspheres 2.0 μm in diameter [42]. It was hypothesized that the particles were picked up by the Kupffer's cells of the liver. Mattrey used perfluoroctylbromide particles 0.5 μm in diameter. This agent produced an increased reflectivity in the liver and spleen, resulting in increased echogenicity usually around the rim of tumors [38]. Recently, iodipamide ethyl ester particles 1 μm in size have been shown to increase the backscatter within the rat liver [46]. Of all the colloidal suspensions the most promising at this point appear to be the perfluorochemicals which are being tested to enhance not only the ultrasound backscatter in tissue but also Doppler signals. In addition, these agents have shown some success in enhancing the attenuation of tissue using X-ray computed tomography [35]. Human experiments are ongoing to demonstrate effectiveness in a variety of areas. In the United States animal as well as human research has shown that it can enhance liver tumors after 24–48 h and, more recently, has been shown to enhance Doppler signals from the blood. Preliminary results have also shown that the agent increases tissue reflectivity of the collecting system of rabbit kidneys [36].

The reflectivity of perfluorocarbons is felt to be due to their high density (1.9 g/ml) and low acoustic velocity (600 mm/s), resulting in an acoustic impedence difference of 30 % between it and the adjacent tissues. Since the impedence difference determines the strength of an echo, perflourocarbons increase the echogenicity of the blood and tissues [35]. The greater the amount given, the greater is the enhancement. For instance, using VX-2 produced tumors in rabbit kidneys, it has been shown that these hypovascular tumors appear less echogenic relative to the normal kidney after injection of this agent. The same effect has been seen in liver tumors, where the reflectivity of the normal tissue is increased relative to less vascular tumors. It should be pointed out that the reverse can occur on occasion, that is, an echogenic liver tumor can appear to become isoechogenic after injection of perfluorochemicals. This is the "vanishing tumor" effect that has been reported in computed tomography, where the difference between normal tissue and tumor is reduced after the injection of an iodinated contrast agent because of relative uptake of the agent in the tissue so that the attenuation between the normal and abnormal tissue becomes equal. The effectiveness of this agent appears to be due to its uptake by the reticuloendothelial system, with the effect increasing over several days. Perflourochemicals have also been shown to enhance Doppler signals in both large and small blood vessels. The agent appears to be removed from the blood either by phagocytosis through the reticuloendothelial system and/or by evaporation through the lung over several days. It should be pointed out that some adverse effects have been shown, including low back pain that was reversible when the infusion rate was reduced. Fever and trembling have also been noted, regressing spontaneously over several hours [35].

Initial research using iodipamide ethyl ester has shown its potential usefulness for enhancing ultrasound images of the liver. These small-diameter particles permit intravenous injection followed by rapid accumulation in the reticuloendothelial system in the liver and spleen. It appears to be distributed throughout the normal liver rather than in tumors. Preliminary investigations suggest that the ultrasound attenuation can be controlled by the choice of the ultrasound frequency, particle concentration, and size. These results, however, have been successful up to now only in animal experiments, and further work is needed before full potential in humans is realized [46].

Numerous approaches have been tried in an attempt to encapsulate or trap gas bubbles. One of the first was the use of hydrogen gas trapped in gelatin capsules. The success of this approach was limited due to the 80-μm size of the particles. However, Carroll was able to show enhancement of tumor rims in rabbits with VX-2 tumor. Injections of this material had to be made directly into an artery, perfusing the area of interest, since the particles would become trapped in the capillary system when it was injected peripherally [7].

Air-filled human albumin has been shown to transverse the pulmonary circulation to increase the reflectivity of blood within the left atrium and ventricle. It has also been shown to pass through the capillary system and result in enhancement of the Doppler signal from various systemic arteries

[26]. These stable, air-filled human albumin microspheres (Albunex) are 1–8 μm (mean 3.8±2.5 μm) in diameter. The half-life of this contrast agent, when injected into blood, has been shown to be less than 1 min. After 3 min more than 80% of the contrast agent was found in the liver. These microspheres are phagocytized by the reticuloendothelial system, with by-products returned to the blood and within 24 hours excreted in the urine [31].

Recent investigations using naturally occurring hepatocellular tumors in woodchucks have shown that intravenous injections of Albunex produced immediate Doppler signal enhancement within the inferior vena cava, followed by enhancement within the abdominal aorta, hepatic artery, and its branches. While the two-dimensional ultrasound images showed no perceivable change in tissue reflectivity of the normal parenchyma, tumor, or vessels, using Doppler (both spectral or color) there was clear signal enhancement. This effect was found in both normal and tumor vessels. The greatest increase in Doppler intensity was apparent at the tumor periphery since the central portion tended to be less vascular and in some cases was necrotic and, thus, enhanced Doppler signals (either color or spectral) were not seen within the central portion of the tumor (Fig. 10). The contrast agent effect increased in proportion to the dose (Fig. 11) [21].

Abnormal blood flow associated with hepatocellular carcinomas, renal carcinomas and breast tumors can be detected with the use of Doppler techniques [47, 55, 59]. With small malignant breast tumors, low signal strength from moving scatterers (blood cells) is "diluted" by that of the adjacent stationary solid tissue, which is a limiting factor in the detection of these small tumors [6]. Ultrasound contrast agents should increase our ability to detect smaller vessels. The results of this preliminary study suggest that air-filled albumin enhances backscatter in both tumor and normal vessels. The ability to detect the motion of blood in small vessels is usually limited in deep tissue by the intensity at the skin surface of the echoes from blood. By increasing this intensity, an intravenously injected contrast agent enables better detection of blood flow in small, deep vessels than is now possible with conventional Doppler techniques. For instance, signals enhanced by contrast agent were detected within woodchuck hepatocellular tumors from vessels that were not detected before the injection of the ultrasound contrast agent. These experiments also suggest that an ultrasound contrast agent would help to differentiate areas of normal vascularity from areas of reduced or absent flow due to the presence of tumor necrosis. The demonstration of normal parenchymal arterial flow within areas that were considered abnormal may help to distinguish tumors from pseudotumors, such as renal columns of Bertin. Ultrasound contrast agents may also enhance echoes from arterial blood and aid in the detection of ischemia or occlusion. In cases of partial occlusion the flow is often fast enough for normal Doppler detection. However, the quantity of blood, which with tissue attenuation determines the signal strength passing through the narrowing, may not be great enough to be detected with current Doppler equipment. Under certain circumstances, the

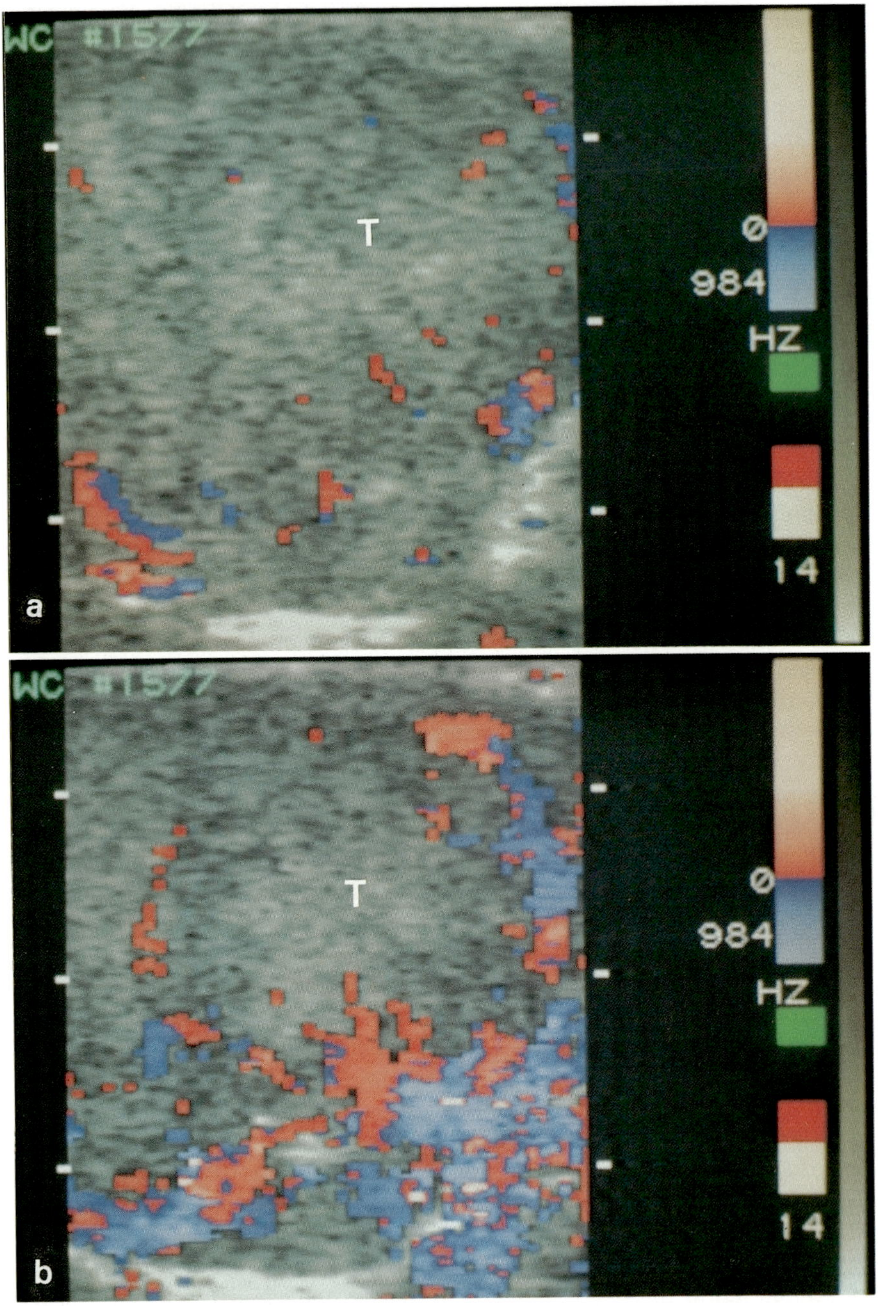

Fig. 10 a, b. The differences in the color Doppler signal just before **(a)** and then after **(b)** the injection of air-filled albumin on the color signal enhancement around a woodchuck hepatocellular tumor *(T)* is clearly seen. At autopsy, the central area of the tumor was found to be undergoing necrosis. (From [21] with permission)

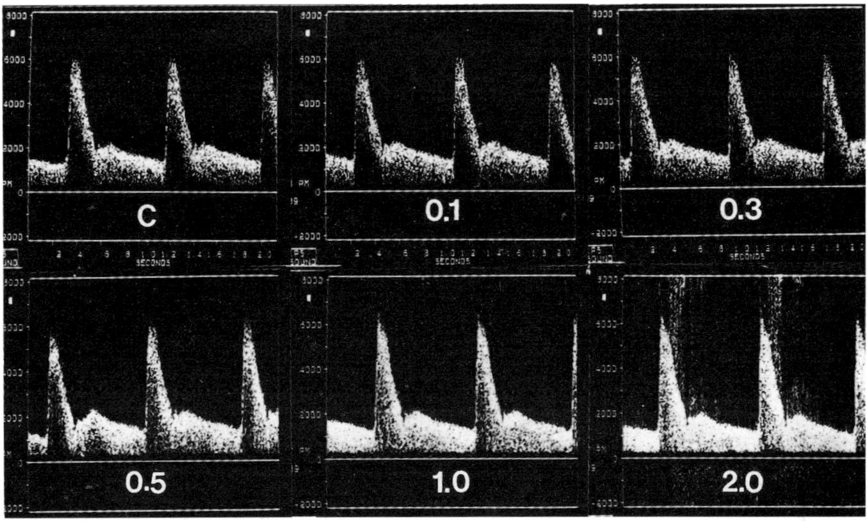

Fig. 11. The spectral measurements obtained from the celiac artery with increasing intravenous doses (0.1–2.0 ml) of air-filled human albumin clearly show progressive increase in the signal intensity. *C*, control. (From [21] with permission)

introduction of more reflectors could aid in the delineation of the site of narrowing. The contrast agent may also aid in the visualization of collaterals caused by occlusion or severe stenosis. While human studies are taking place using these gas-containing albumin particles to evaluate cardiac chambers and myocardial infusion, other areas await Food and Drug Administration approval before further human research can commence [31].

One of the problems with ultrasound contrast agents has been inadequate standardization in terms of concentration, size and stability. An attempt to solve these problems was made with the development of soluble saccharide (galactose) microparticles containing microbubbles of gas (SHU-454) [15]. These microparticles have a medium diameter of 3.5 μm, with 99 % smaller than 12 μm. Trials were carried out in both animals and humans in which contrast injected intravenously was imaged ultrasonically in the right atrium and ventricle. However, since the bubble sizes in suspension range from 5 to 15 μm, they could not easily pass from the right to the left side of the heart. This agent, however, can be used when directly injected into arteries to visualize the organs that they are perfusing [40]. For instance, when injected into flowing blood, the contrast agent could be readily visualized with both two-dimensional ultrasound imaging and Doppler (both spectral and color). When injected into the arterial supply of organs such as the kidney, this contrast material produced enhanced visualization of small vessels within the organ, producing a capillary blush seen on color Doppler imaging as well as improving the signal-to-noise ratio of the Doppler signals obtained from vessels within this organ. While this research was performed in animals, it shows promise for applications in humans. A limitation of this agent, however, is that it cannot be injected into a peripheral vein and still produce an effect in vessels and organs beyond the heart. More recently, a new monosaccharide agent SHU-508 has been produced to image the left side of the heart [52, 53]. This agent is made from galactose but is produced with a slight change in its chemical composition to produce smaller, more uniform bubble sizes 2–8 μm in diameter, with 97 % of the bubbles measuring less than 6 μm. Thus, this agent has been used successfully to visualize not only the right but also the left side of the heart. In addition, it is a nontoxic, neutral ph, biodegradable agent which is made from a naturally occurring substance. The agent appears useful in delineating the circumference of the chambers of the heart as well as in assisting in the calculation of ventricular ejection fraction. It should also prove useful in visualizing, as well as quantifying, left-to-right shunts and it has the potential for producing myocardial enhancement, although more research is needed in this area [52].

As the result of its ability to transverse the cardiopulmonary circulation, we have evaluated SHU-508 in noncardiac areas of the body. In animal studies peripheral intravenous injections have resulted in enhancement of the Doppler signal (both spectral and color) in major vessels throughout the body. Enhancement of smaller vessels in both the liver and the kidneys has also been documented. Of more interest is its ability to enhance Doppler signals in the portal circulation, which means the contrast agent passed through two capillary beds. In addition, there is evidence of recirculation of this agent, although at decreased concentrations. Research with naturally occurring hepatocellular carcinomas in woodchucks has confirmed its ability to increase the reflectivity of small vessels not only within the normal portions of the liver but also within the tumors (Fig. 12). There was increasing effect with increasing dose. The ultrasound contrast effects have also been demonstrated in the celiac artery in woodchucks at doses as small as 0.025 ml/kg. This agent, thus, shows promise of becoming an important new ultrasound contrast agent with an effectiveness similar to that of computed tomography and angiographic radiologic contrast agents.

Besides the use of ultrasound contrast agents via intraarterial or intravenous injections, research has also shown the feasibility of using these agents to improve visualization of the fallopian tube. Contrast agents have been introduced through catheters placed within the cervical os. Increased reflectivity (echogenicity) was seen within both the perfused fallopian tube and the endometrial cavity [10]. However, initial results have shown no significant improvement over hysteroscopy or hysterosalpingography [9]. More work in this area is needed before its efficacy can be fully established. This ultrasound contrast agent has also been placed within the urinary bladder in an attempt to visualize reflux into the ureters, with limited success. Injection, through needles, of a small amount of microbubble-containing material has been used to improve ultrasound-guided biopsy or drainage procedures.

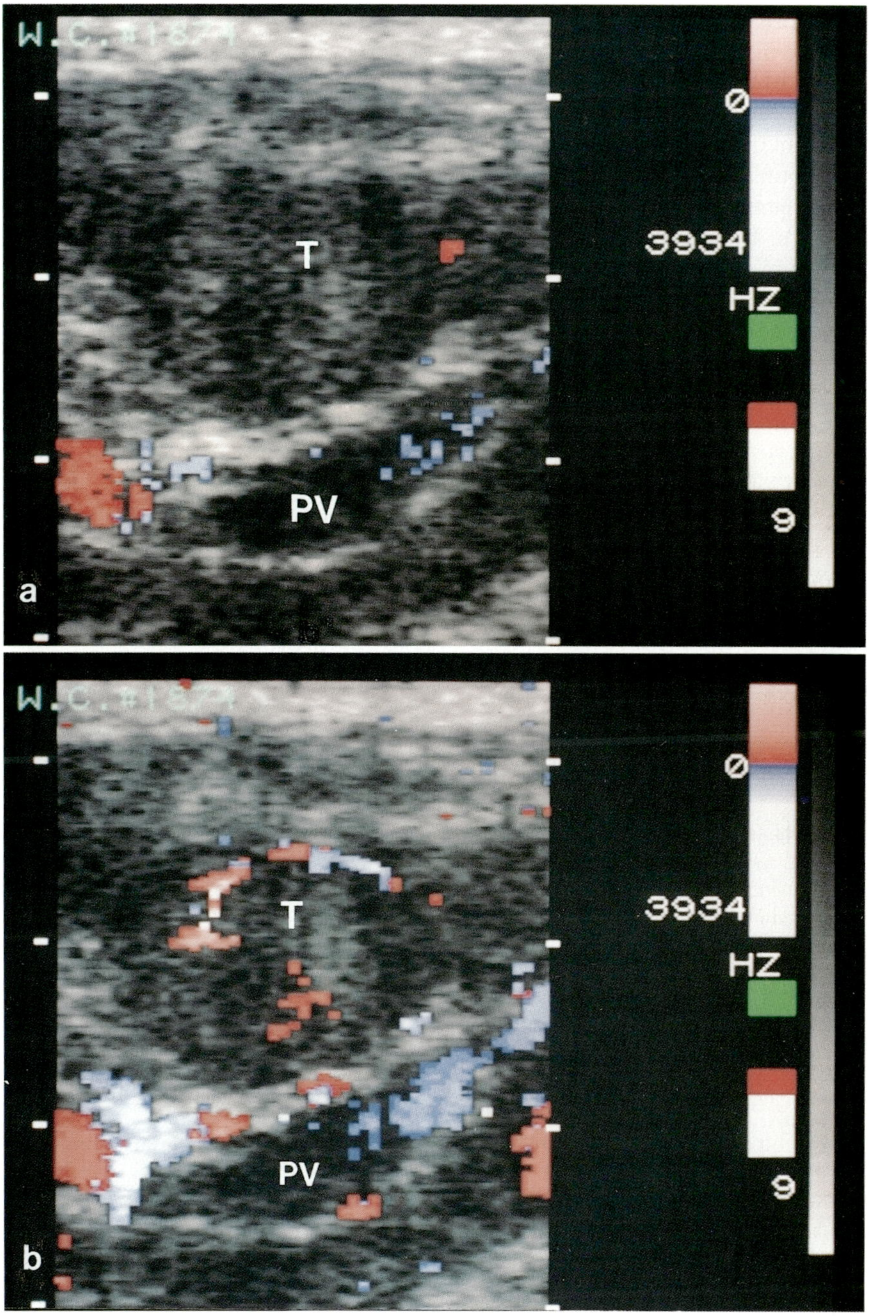

Fig. 12a, b. Color Doppler signal enhancement is seen within a woodchuck hepatocellular tumor *(T)* before **(a)** and after **(b)** intravenous injection of an air-containing sugar complex (SHU-508). *PV,* portal vein

Summary

It should be pointed out that for radiologic applications, the most effective contrast agents are those that pass through the pulmonary bed and heart and still remain intact in sufficient concentration to enhance the backscattered ultrasound signal. For noncardiac diagnosis, the ideal ultrasound contrast agent would be nontoxic, injectable intravenously, and capable of passing through the pulmonary capillary and cardiac circulations to enhance detection of blood flowing in small vessels. A variety of potential ultrasound contrast agents have been or are now under development. Preliminary results in animals and limited research in humans suggest that ultrasound contrast agents will become commercially available in the not too distant future.

Acknowledgements. We wish to thank the following who have worked with us on one or more of the research projects discussed in this chapter: Archie A. Alexander, M.D., Demetrius H. Bagley, M.D., Peter N. Burns, Ph.D., Herbert E. Cohn, M.D., Rick I. Feld, M.D., Thomas G. Helinek, M.D., Kathleen Kuhlman, M.D., Alfred B. Kurtz, M.D., Barbara McComb, M.D., Daniel A. Merton, B.S., R.D.M.S., Larry S. Miller, M.D., Laurence Needleman, M.D., Bruce E. Northrup, M.D., David S. Prince, M.D., Marcelle J. Shapiro, M.D., and Jerome J. Vearnick, M.D.

References

1. Becher H, Schlief R, Lüderitz B (1989) Improved sensitivity of color Doppler by SHU 454. Am J Cardiol 64: 374
2. Berwing K, Schlepper M (1988) Echocardiographic imaging of the left ventricle by peripheral intravenous injection of echocontrast agent. Am Heart J 115: 339–408
3. Bom N, Lancee CT, van Egmond FC (1972) An ultrasonic intracardiac scanner. Ultrasonics 10: 72–76
4. Bommer WJ, Shah P, Allen H, Meltzer R, Kisslo J (1984) Contrast echocardiography. Report of the American Society of Echocardiography, pp 1–10
5. Botet JF, Lightdale C (1991) Endoscopic sonography of the upper gastrointestinal tract. AJR Am J Roentgenol 156: 63–68
6. Burns PN, Halliwell M, Wells PNT, Webb AJ (1982) Ultrasonic Doppler studies of the breast. Ultrasound Med Biol 8: 127–143
7. Carroll BA, Turner RJ, Tickner EG, Boyle DB, Young SW (1980) Gelatin encapsulated nitrogen microbubbles as ultrasonic contrast agents. Invest Radiol 15/3: 260–266
8. Carroll BA, Turner R, Tichner G. Young SW (1979) Microbubbles as ultrasonic contrast agents. Invest Radiol 14/5: 374
9. Deichert U, Schlief R, van de Sandt M, Juhnke I (1989) Transvaginal hysterosalpingo-contrast-sonography (Hy-Co-Sy) compared with conventional tubal diagnostics. Hum Reprod 4/4: 418–424
10. Deichert U, van de Sandt M, Lauth G, Daume E (1988) Die transvaginale Hysterokontrastsonographie (HKSG). Geburtshilfe Frauenheilkd 48: 835–844
11. Feigenbaum H, Stone J, Lee D et al. (1970) Identification of ultrasound echoes from the left ventricle by use of intracardiac injections of indocine green. Circulation 41: 615–621

12. Feinstein SB, Shah PM, Bing RJ et al. (1984) Microbubble dynamics visualized in the intact capillary circulation. J Am Coll Cardiol 4/3: 595–600
13. Feinstein SB, TenCate FJ, Zwehl W et al. (1984) Two-dimensional contrast echocardiography. I. In vitro development and quantitative analysis of echo contrast agents. J Am Coll Cardiol 3/1: 14–20
14. Fink IJ, Miller DJ, Shawker TH (1985) Lipid emulsions as contrast agents for hepatic sonography: an experimental study in rabbits. Ultrason Imaging 7: 191–197
15. Fritzsch T, Schartl M, Siegert J (1988) Preclinical and clinical results with an ultrasonic contrast agent. Invest Radiol 23 [Suppl 1]: S302 – S305
16. Fukuda M, Hirata K, Saito K et al. (1980) On the diagnostic use of echoendoscope in abdominal disease. I. Diagnostic experiences with a new type of echoendoscope on gastric diseases. Proc Jpn J Med Ultrasound 37: 409–410
17. Gillam LD, Kaul S, Fallon JT, Levine RA, Hedley-Whyte ET, Guerrero JL, Weyman AE (1984) Functional and pathologic effects of multiple echocardiographic contrast injections on the myocardium, brain and kidney. J Am Coll Cardiol 6/3: 687–694
18. Goldberg BB (1971) Ultrasonic measurement of the aortic arch, right pulmonary artery, and left atrium. Radiology 101/2: 383–390
19. Goldberg BB (1976) Ultrasonic cholangiography, gray-scale B-scan evaluation of the common bile duct. Radiology 118: 401–404
20. Goldberg BB, Bagley D, Liu JB et al. (1991) Endoluminal sonography of the urinary tract: preliminary observations. Am J Roentgenol 156: 99–103
21. Goldberg BB, Hilpert P, Burns P et al. (1990) Hepatic tumors: signal enhancement of Doppler US after intravenous injection of a contrast agent. Radiology 177: 713–717
22. Goldberg BB, Liu JB, Merton DA et al. (1990) Endoluminal US: experiments with nonvascular uses in animals. Radiology 175: 39–43
23. Goldberg BB, Liu JB, Kuhlmann K et al. (1991) Endoluminal gynecologic ultrasound: preliminary results. J Ultrasound Med 10: 583–590
24. Gramiak R, Shah PM (1968) Echocardiography of the aortic root. Invest Radiol 3: 356–366
25. Heyder N (1987) Endoscopic ultrasonography of tumours of the oesophagus and the stomach. Surg Endosc 1: 17–23
26. Hilpert PL, Mattrey RF, Mitten RM, Peterson T (1989) IV injection of air-filled human albumin microspheres to enhance arterial Doppler signal: a preliminary study in rabbits. Am J Roentgenol 153: 613–616
27. Holm HH, Northeved AA (1974) A transurethral ultrasonic scanner. J Urol 111: 238–248
28. Isner JM, Rosenfield K, Losordo DW et al. (1990) Percutaneous intravascular US as adjunct to catheter-based interventions: preliminary experience in patients with peripheral vascular disease. Radiology 175: 61–70
29. Keller MW, Feinstein SB, Briller RA, Powsner SM (1986) Automated production and analysis of echo contrast agents. J Ultrasound Med 5: 493–498
30. Keller MW, Feinstein SB, Watson DD (1987) Successful left ventricular opacification following peripheral venous injection of sonicated contrast agent: an experimental evaluation. Am Heart J 114: 570–575
31. Keller MW, Glasheen W, Kaul S (1989) Albunex: a safe and effective commercially produced agent for myocardial contrast echocardiography. J Am Soc Echocardiology 2: 48–52
32. Kerber RE, Kioschos JM, Lauer RM (1974) Use of an ultrasonic contrast method in the diagnosis of valvular regurgitation and intracardiac shunts. Am J Cardiol 34: 722–727
33. Lang RM, Feinstein SB, Feldman T, Neumann A, Chua KG, Borow KM (1986) Contrast echocardiography for evaluation of myocardial perfusion: effects of coronary angioplasty. J Am Coll Cardiol 8: 232–235
34. Mallery JA, Gregory K, Morcos NC et al. (1987) Evaluation of an ultrasound balloon dilatation imaging catheter. Circulation 76 [Suppl IV]: 371

35. Mattrey RF (1989) Perfluorooctylbromide: a new contrast agent for CT, sonography, and MR imaging. Am J Roentgenol 152: 247–252
36. Mattrey RF, Mitten R, Peterson T, Long CD (1987) Vascular ultrasonic enhancement of tissues with perfluorooctylbromide for renal tumor detection. Radiology 165 [Suppl]: 76 (abstr)
37. Mattrey RF, Scheible FW, Gosink BB, Leopold GR, Long DM, Higgins CB (1982) Perfluorooctylbromide: a liver/spleen-specific and tumor-imaging ultrasound contrast material. Radiology 145: 759–762
38. Mattrey RF, Strich G, Shelton RE et al. (1987) Perfluorochemicals in US contrast agents for tumor imaging and hepatosplenography: preliminary clinical results. Radiology 163: 339–343
39. Meyer CR, Chiang EH, Fechner KP et al. (1988) Feasibility of high-resolution, intravascular ultrasonic imaging catheters. Radiology 168: 113–116
40. Mouaaouy AE, Becker HD, Schlief R, Kuhlo C, Portas C (1990) Rat liver model for testing intraoperative echo contrast sonography. Surg Endosc 4: 114–117
41. Murata Y, Suzuki S, Hashimoto H (1988) Endoscopic ultrasonography of the upper gastrointestinal tract. Surg Endosc 2: 180–183
42. Ophir J, Gobuty A, McWhirt RE, Maklad NF (1980) Ultrasonic backscatter from contrast producing collagen microspheres. Ultrason Imaging 2: 67–77
43. Ophir J, McWhirt RE, Maklad NF (1979) Aqueous solutions as potential ultrasonic contrast agents. Ultrason Imaging 1: 265–279
44. Ophir J, Parker KJ (1989) Contrast agents in diagnostic ultrasound. Ultrasound Med Biol 15/4: 319–333
45. Pandian NG, Kreis A, Brockway B et al. (1988) Ultrasound angioscopy: real-time, two-dimensional, intraluminal ultrasound imaging of blood vessels. Am J Cardiol 62: 493–494
46. Parker KJ, Tuthill TA, Lerner RM, Violante MR (1987) A particulate contrast agent with potential for ultrasound imaging of liver. Ultrasound Med Biol 13/9: 555–566
47. Ramos I, Taylor KJW, Kier R, Burns PN, Snower DP, Carter D (1988) Tumor vascular signals in renal masses: detection with Doppler US. Radiology 168: 633–637
48. Reid CL, Kawanishi DT, McKay CR et al. (1983) Accuracy of evaluation of the presence and severity of aortic and mitral regurgitation by contrast 2-dimensional echocardiography. Am J Cardiol 52: 519
49. Reisner SA, Shapiro JR, Schwarz KQ, Meltzer RS (1988) Sonication of echo-contrast agents: a standardized and reproducible method. J Cardiovasc Ultrasonogr 7/3: 273–276
50. Rosch T, Lorenz R, Braig C, Feuerbach S, Siewert JR, Classen M (1990) Endosonographische Diagnostik bei Pankreastumoren. Dtsch Med Wochenschr 115: 1339–1347
51. Sahn DJ, Valdez-Cruz LM (1984) Ultrasonic contrast studies for the detection of cardiac shunts. J Am Coll Cardiol 3: 978
52. Schlief R, Staks T, Mahler M, Rufer M, Fritzsch T, Seifert W (1990) Successful opacification of the left heart chambers on echocardiographic examination after intravenous injection of a new saccharide based contrast agent. Echocardiography 7/1: 61–64
53. Smith MD, Elion JL, McClure RR et al. (1989) Left heart opacification with peripheral venous injection of a new saccharide echo contrast agent in dogs. J Am Coll Cardiol 13/7: 1622–1628
54. Takada T, Yasuda H, Uchiyama K, Hasegawa H, Shikata J (1990) Contrast-enhanced intraoperative ultrasonography of small hepatocellular carcinomas. Surgery 107: 528–532
55. Taylor KJW, Ramos I, Carter D et al. (1988) Correlation of Doppler US tumor signals with neovascular morphologic features. Radiology 166: 57–62
56. Tei C, Kondo S, Meerbaum S et al. (1984) Correlation of myocardial echo contrast disappearance rate ("washout") and severity of experimental coronary stenosis. J Am Coll Cardiol 3: 39–46

57. Tyler TD, Ophir J, Maklad NF (1981) In vivo enhancement of ultrasonic image luminance by aqueous solutions with high speed of sound. Ultrason Imaging 3: 323–329
58. von Micsky LI (1966) Ultrasonic tomography in obstetrics and gynecology. In: Grossman CC, Holmes JH, Joyner C et al. (eds) Diagnostic ultrasound. Plenum, New York, pp 348–368
59. Wells PNT, Halliwell M, Skidmore R, Webb AJ, Woodcock JP (1977) Tumour detection by ultrasound Doppler blood flow signals. Ultrasonics 15: 231–232
60. Wild JJ, Reid JM (1957) Progress in techniques of soft tissue examination by 15 MC pulsed ultrasound. In: Kelly E (ed) Ultrasound in medicine and biology. American Institute of Biological Science, Washington DC, pp 30–45
61. Yock PG, Linker DT, White NW et al. (1989) Clinical applications of intravascular ultrasound imaging in atherectomy. Int J Card Imaging 4: 117–125
62. Ziskin MC, Bonakdapour A, Weinstein DP, Lynch PR (1972) Contrast agents for diagnostic ultrasound. Invest Radiol 6: 500–505

Possibilities of Three-Dimensional Sonography in Obstetrics

A. Kratochwil

Progress in medical sonography has hitherto come about in response to clinical demands that were answered by engineers on the basis of available technology. Now, for the first time, the development of a new method has been stimulated by engineers, and the clinician must evaluate the practical utility of the new technique.

The purpose of sonography has always been to obtain a three-dimensional image of the examined region of interest. Using usual two-dimensional scans, the examiner tries to obtain a three-dimensional impression of the form, size, and location of a pathological lesion. The reliability of such a procedure is largely dependent on the ability of examiner. A disadvantage is the lack of feedback to the machine and the possibility of a subsequent interpretation.

Various attempts have been made to present sonographic findings in three dimensions, for instance, stereoscopic inspection of the scans, the application of additional mechanical systems to establish volume coordinates, and processing the data by computer systems. The time needed for aquiring and processing the data is in most cases so long as to make an interaction between the machine and the examiner impossible. Some of the methods applied display only the surface of the object under examination. This is, however, a serious drawback to the usual techniques, as sonography is dependent on information derived from the organ structure. Three-dimensional imaging without loss of valuable information is possible if only one scan is performed, and the acquired information is simultaneously displayed in three different planes.

The aim of the three-dimensional Voluson (Kretztechnik, Zipf, Austria) here was:

1) simple, quick, and complete acquisition of a sample volume for three-dimensional interpretation,
2) the production of a sonographic scan containing all relevant information,
3) a system without expensive periphery, and
4) no substantial changes in handling compared to the usual techniques.

To achieve this a 3-MHz annular array transducer scans a tissue pyramid, with the top of the pyramid near the transducer's window (Figs. 1–3). The

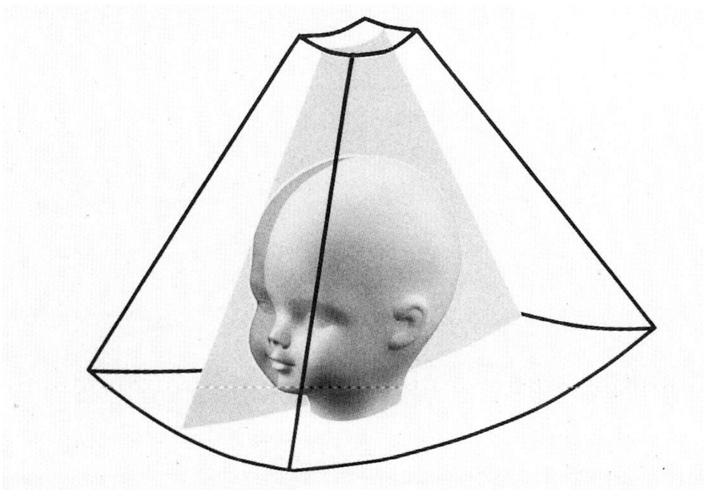

Fig. 1. Volume box with the fetal head, longitudinal scan

scan is performed automatically. By swiveling the transducer a series of scans is stored over 5 s. The standard volume is 18 cm in length, 6 cm in width, and 9 cm in depth. Handling differs from that of the usual system only so far as the region of interest must be placed within the volume box on the monitor. The volume contains, depending on geometry, 64–256 scans per plane. The annular array technique guarantees selected focusing of the transmitter as a dynamic receiver focusing.

The monitor demonstrates sinultaneously three corresponding scans perpendicular to each other. Normally the upper left quadrant of the monitor

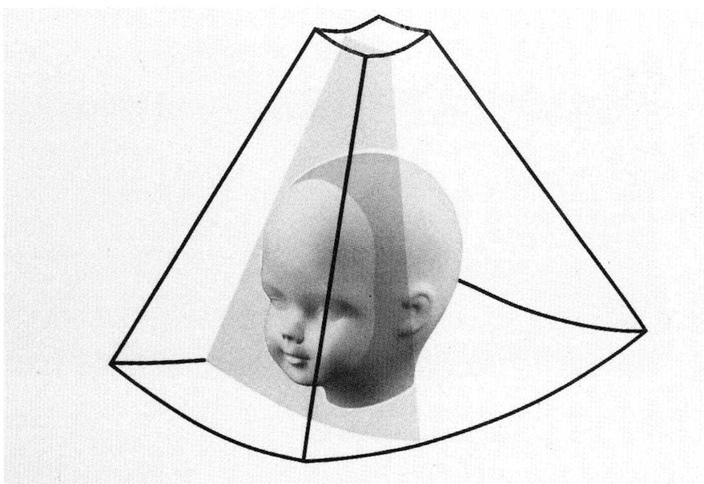

Fig. 2. Volume box with the fetal head, transverse scan

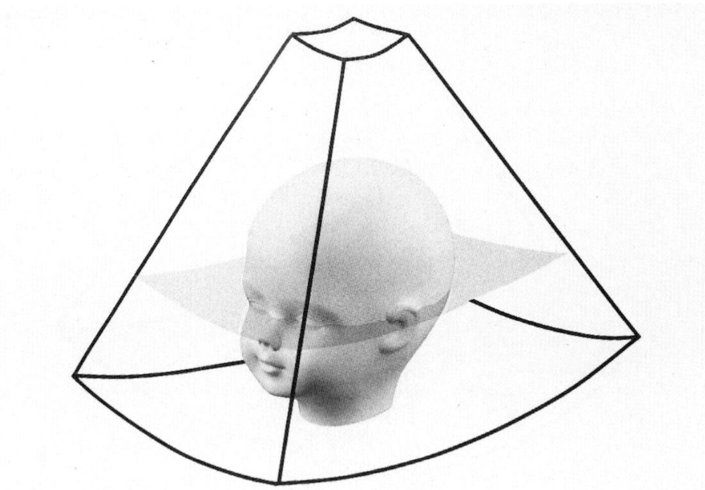

Fig. 3. Volume box with the fetal head, C scan

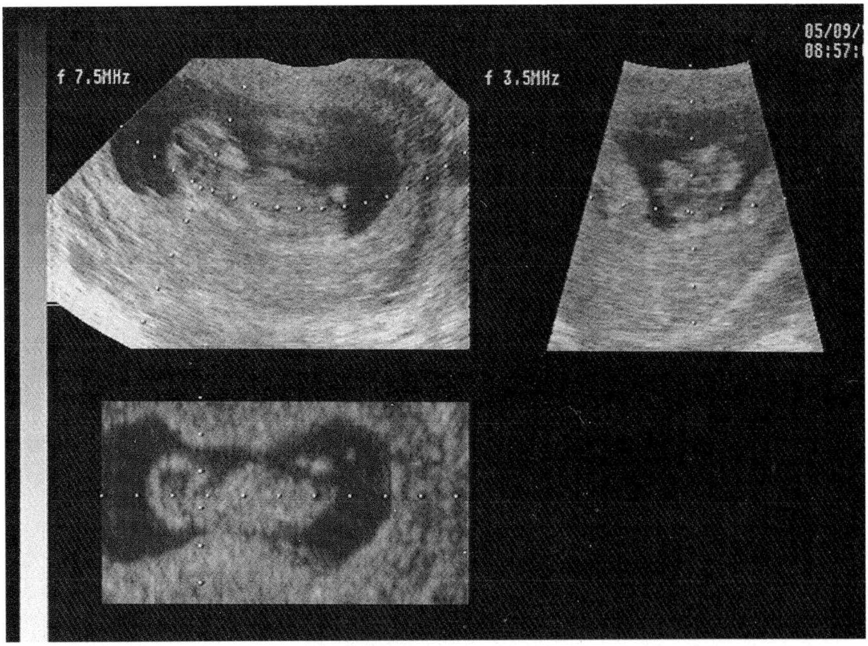

Fig. 4. Pregnancy of 10 weeks. *Upper left,* longitudinal scan; *upper right,* transverse scan; *lower left,* C scan from lateral to medial

shows the longitudinal scan, the upper right the transverse scan, the lower left the C scan, and the lower right the three-dimensional one. The C scan has not been available until now and adds further information. If the examination is started with a longitudinal scan, the C scan presents a horizontal plane from lateral to medial. Starting with a transverse scan, the C scan represents a frontal or coronal plane, which previously could not be presented. Unfortunately, due to physical conditions the quality of resolution of the C scan is below that of the other scans. By calculation the lower right quadrant of the monitor obtains a pseudo-three-dimensional picture.

The stored information allows an interpretation even in the absence of the patient. One can use the stored information in a way similar to turning the pages of a book. Coordinates assist orientation within the stored volume. To guarantee that identical structures are demonstrated in all simultaneously shown scans, the structure is positioned at the coordinate intersection.

Electronic calipers allow distance measurement and the calculation of areas, circumferences, and volumes. Positioning a rectangle, variable in size, within a region-of-interest tissue density is possible in the form of a histiogram.

Documentation is obtained by videotape, hardcopy, or floppy disk. Using a floppy disk not only makes picture interpretation possible at a later period, but also makes it feasible for the patient to be examined later with identical instrument settings.

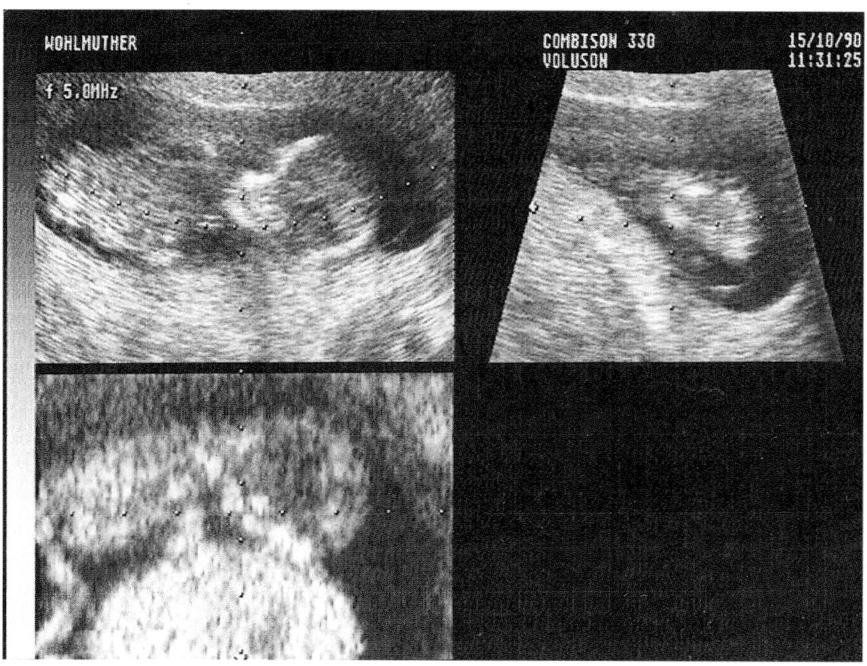

Fig. 5. Pregnancy of 12 weeks. *Lower left,* C scan demonstration of limbs

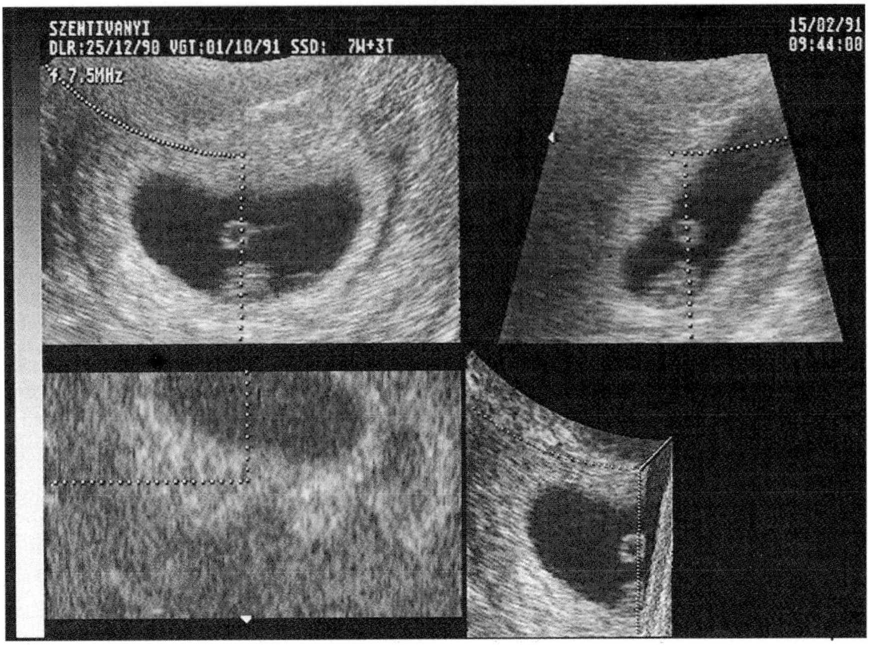

Fig. 6. Pregnancy of 7 weeks, demonstrating the yolk sac. *Lower right,* three-dimensional demonstration

In *pregnancy* a satisfactory demonstration of the fetus is possible up to the 30th week of gestation. At a later stage of pregnancy the demonstration is unsatisfactory as it becomes difficult to place the fetus totally within the volume box. In early pregnancy the fetus can be analyzed in all dimensions. Particularly the C scan improves the demonstration of the limbs a crown-rump measurement (Figs. 4, 5). The yolk sac can be demonstrated in three dimensions (Fig. 6). During the second trimester all fetal structures are satisfactorily demonstrated in all three scans. Especially good demonstration of the intracranial structures can be achieved, such as the corpus callosum and ventricles (Fig. 7). Occasionally the fetal profile can be depicted. As mentioned above, the C scan gives additional information. Starting the examination with a transverse scan through the fetal body, a frontal of coronar scan can be achieved, and layer-per-layer from one to the opposite the abdominal wall can be demonstrated (Fig. 8). The picture is shown in the upper left quadrant the transverse scan of the fetal abdomen; in the upper right the longitudinal scan is shown. The C scan, over left, demonstrates the fetal spine, and in front of it the fetal aorta with its arc and the fetal heart. Within all three scans the crossing of the coordinates is positioned within the aortic vessel. A new aspect of organ relations may influence malformation diagnosis. Figure 9 demonstrates a meningocele in three different scans with the coordinates placed at the solid part within the cystic lesion.

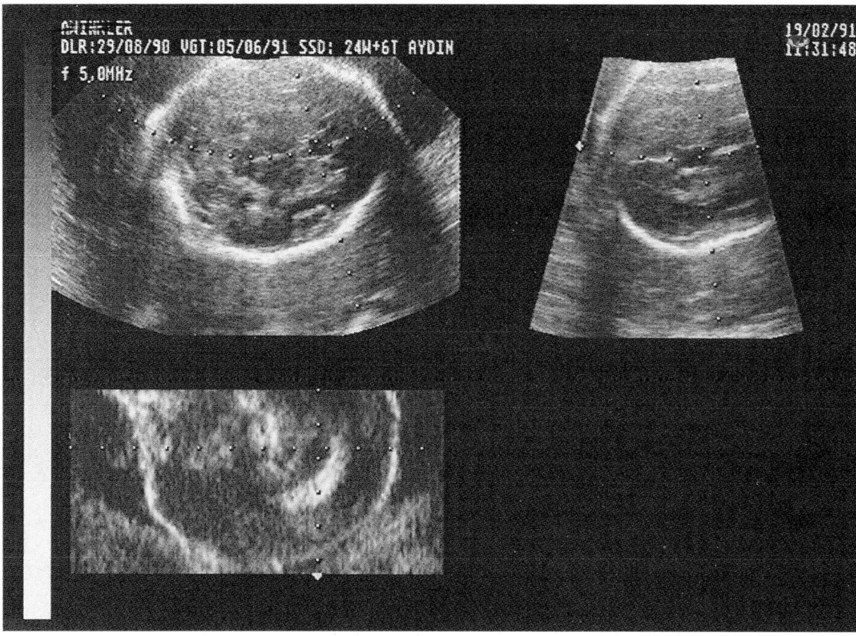

Fig. 7. Pregnancy of 24 weeks, fetal skull. *Lower left,* corpus callosum. Intersection of coordinates within cavum septi pellucidi

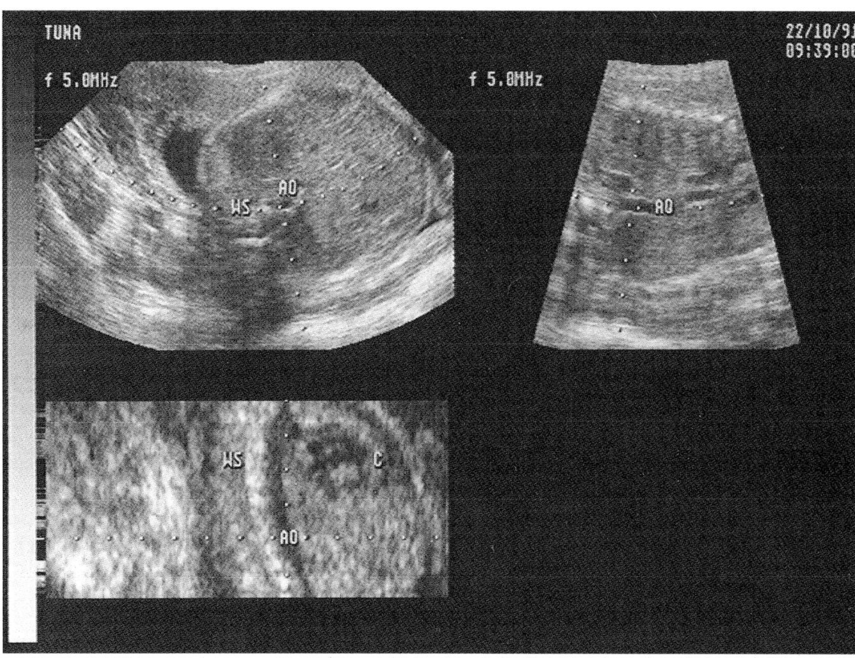

Fig. 8. Demonstration of the fetal aorta

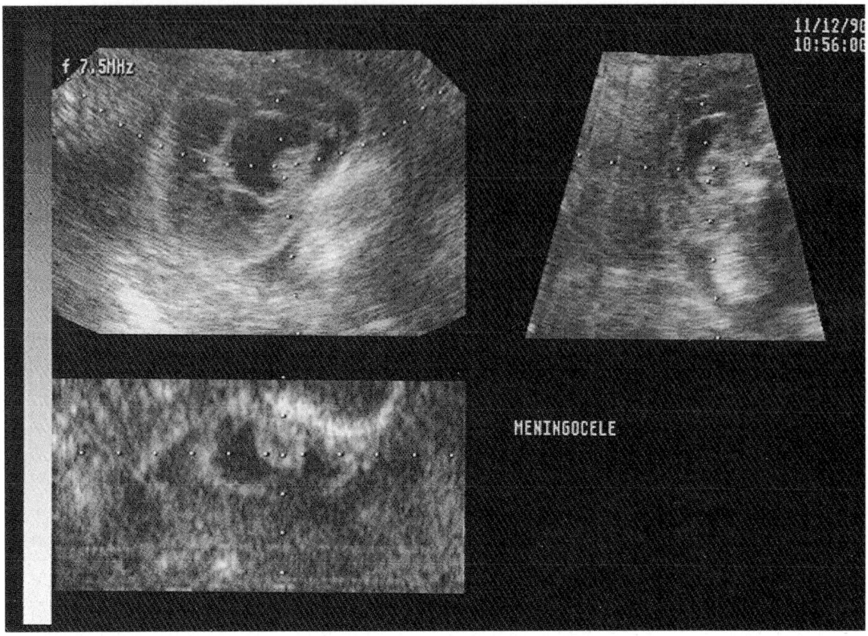

Fig. 9. Meningocele with solid parts

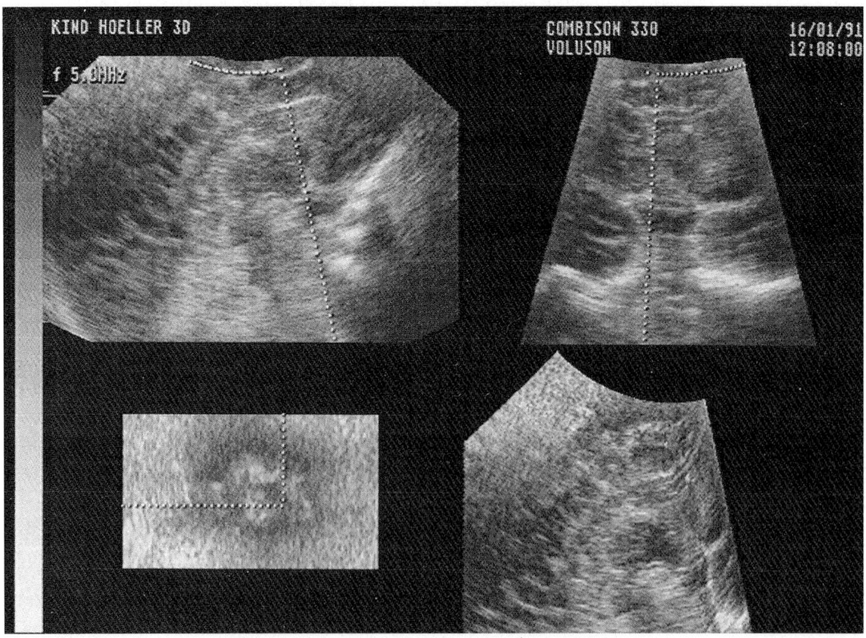

Fig. 10. Postpartal scan of the skull

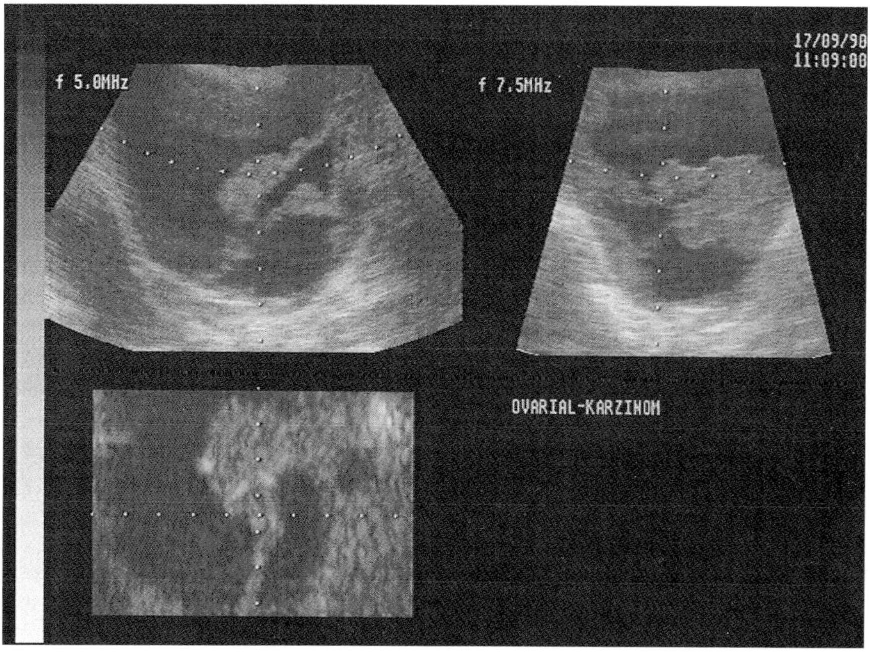

Fig. 11. Carcinoma of the ovary with septa and solid parts

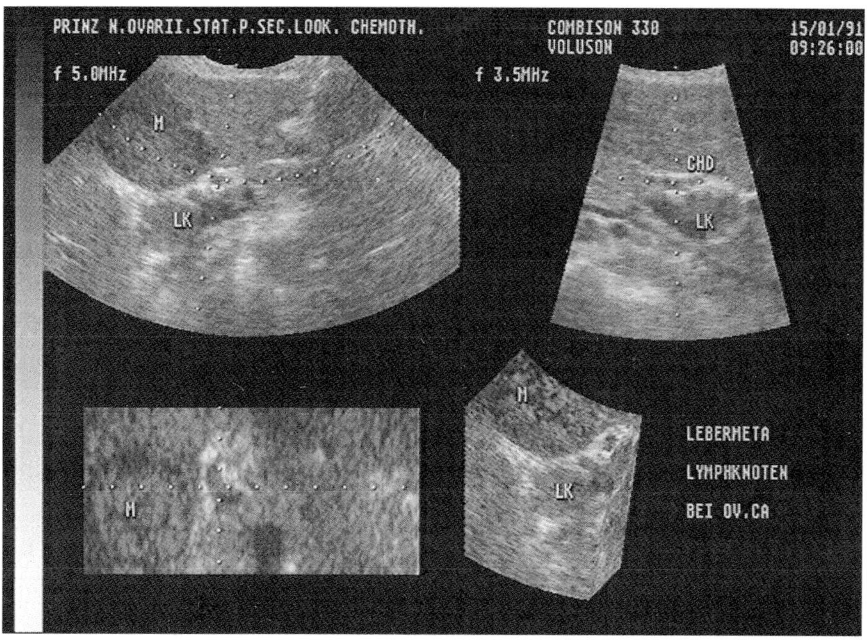

Fig. 12. Involvement of liver and lymph nodes in ovarian carcinoma. *M*, Metastais; *LK*, lymph node; *CHD*, common bile duct, coordinates within the common bile duct

In *postpartal* life this technique can be successfully integrated in the diagnosis and localization of intracranial lesions. By the simultaneous demonstration of all three scans identification of intracranial structures, such as ventricles, thalami, and plexus is substantially improved and is much easier than previously. Figure 10 shows a scan of the fetal skull, demonstrating corpus callosum and ventricles, including the 4th ventricle.

In *gynecology* the three-dimensional technique is of advantage in analyzing genital tumors, particularly of ovarian masses (Fig. 11). This is also the case for the examination of the upper abdomen. Location and spread of paraortic lymph nodes and liver involvement, especially the relationship to the vessels inside the organ, can be demonstrated more clearly than before (Fig. 12). A further improvement can be expected in connection with Doppler methods in placing the Doppler gate even in smaller vessels.

We are certainly standing at the cradle of a new technique. In spite of all present shortcomings the future of this baby promises to be a bright one.

Three-Dimensional Volumetric Scans: Acquisition Technique and Volume Content Viewing

A. Hesse

The three-dimensional (3-D) presentation of organs, tumors, and tissue structures is used routinely with data from computed tomography (CT) and magnetic resonance imaging (MRI). In both procedures sequences of parallel two-dimensional (2-D) slices are acquired. This information can be reconstructed into 3-D presentations by means of digital image processing. The main disadvantages of these procedures are long acquisition time and, with respect to CT, the administration of ionizing radiation. Both methods are very complex, expensive, and not readily available as a routinely used imaging tool. Furthermore, the application in fetal diagnostics is not recommended. Sonography, with its well-known advantages of fast handling, maximum patient safety, and vast availability, shows a promise as a basis for 3-D presentation. Of course, we must take into account the poorer geometrical resolution compared to CTand MRI, although high-end echographic systems today are able to offer very good performance with resolutions below 1 mm.

Recent advances in microprocessor and software technology allow a cost-effective approach to 3-D sonography within a price range that appears acceptable to the users of high-end medical ultrasound equipment. (For an excellent review of the status and perspective of 3-D echography see [1]).

This chapter describes a possible approach to transducer technology and 3-D presentation that has resulted in some initial clinical prototypes. Figure 1 presents the various modules of our current prototype setup. The ultrasound images are acquired in standard 2-D mode using conventional ultrasound equipment (Dornier AI 3200). The prototype 3-D workstation consists of a PC-based microprocessor system with an 80486 processor, 16 Mbytes of random access memory (RAM), a VGA graphics board, a hard disk drive and optional magneto-optical disk drive (MO), a 16-in. color monitor, a frame grabber to digitize the ultrasound video signal, and a coprocessor unit based on Intel's 1860 RISC processor. In addition, connected to the 3-D workstation and to the ultrasound unit via the transducer is a stepper motor control unit for the positioning of the transducer array inside the 3-D scanhead. The currently used frame grabber will be replaced by a LAN interface for strictly digital data transfer in all future applications. This will reduce costs in addition to assuring minimum information loss through direct transfer of digital data from the ultrasound unit scan converter to the digital PC memory.

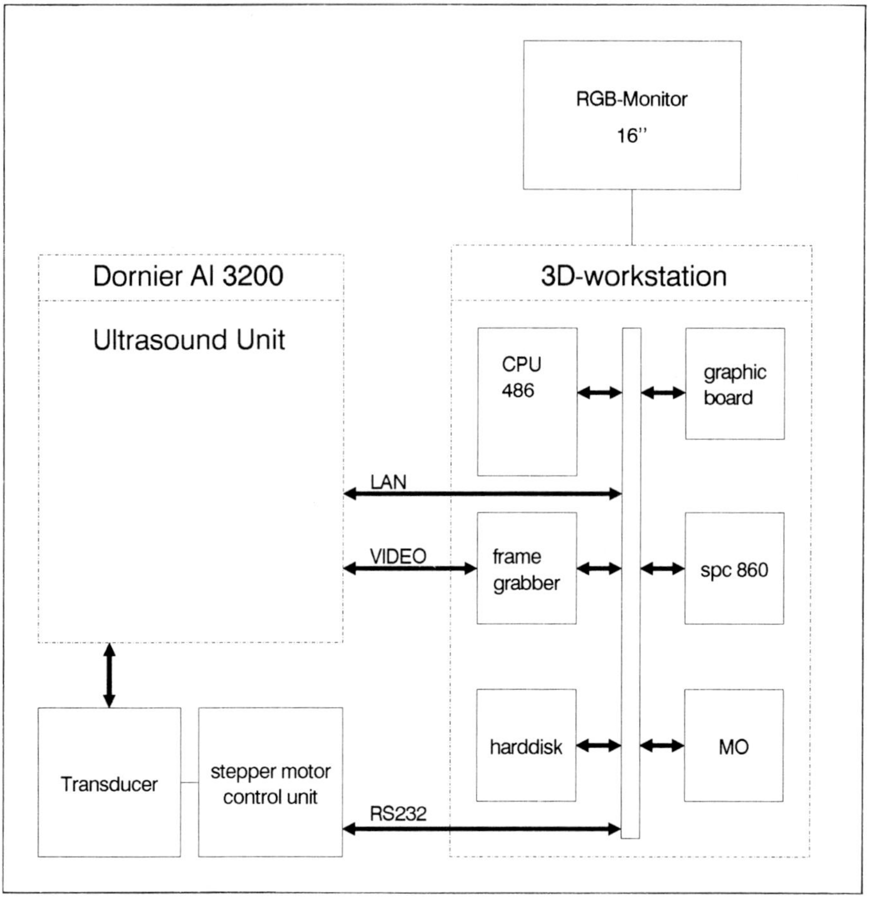

Fig. 1. Block diagram of clinical prototype

The custom-built 3-D scanhead presented here features a curved linear array transducer which can be swiveled ±30° from its center position (Fig. 2). Precise positioning of the transducer array is achieved by a stepper motor mounted inside the transducer handle (Fig. 3). Throughout the acquisition of the volume scan the single 2-D slices can be controlled on the monitor of the ultrasound system. The complete handling of the 3-D workstation during data acquisition is controlled by two switches located at the transducer handle, thus allowing manipulation of the scanhead to be performed similarly to a standard diagnostic procedure. This occurs without additional user action concerning the 3-D workstation (e.g., keyboard inputs).

The principle of swiveling the transducer over the user-selectable angle within ±30° was chosen to avoid the acquisition of redundant data as it appears, with scanheads, where the transducer is rotated around the central image axis during data acquisition. In addition to choosing the appropriate

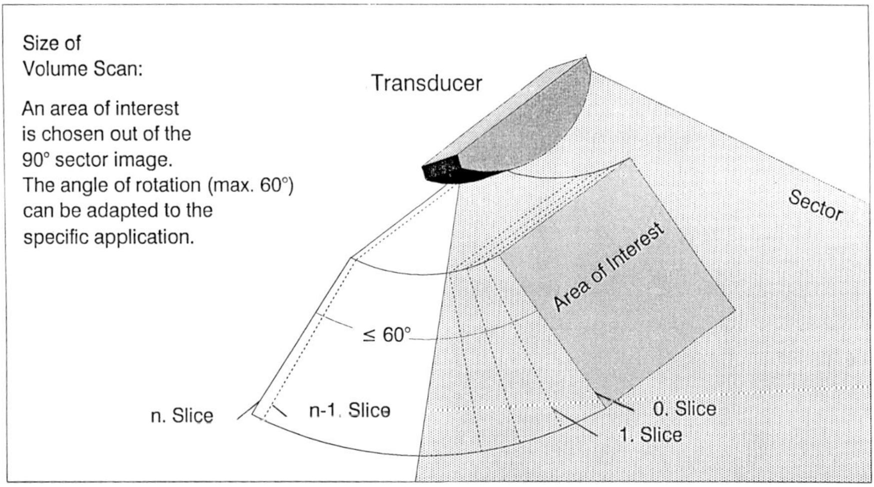

Fig. 2. Principle of transducer movement to perform volume scan

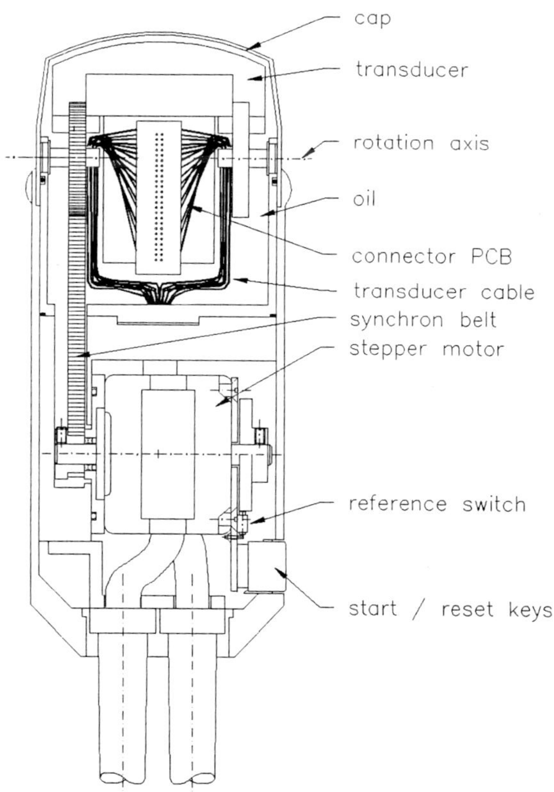

Fig. 3. Schematic drawing of 3-D transducer

sweep angle, the number of images acquired (and there by the spacing between individual slices) can be selected by the user.

The resolution of the scanned volume can be adapted to the specific diagnostic application by varying these parameters. The size of the chosen sweep angle and the number of images acquired within this angle determine the time necessary to record one volume scan. Depending on the frame rate of the ultrasound system used (the frame rate depends mainly on penetration depth and the kind of focusing applied), a typical time to record one volumetric scan is around 10 s. Clinical trials have shown that a comfortable data acquisition free of artifacts can be performed within such a period using a hand-held 3-D scanhead in the abdominal area, where no periodical variations or tissue movements are to be expected.

The transducer array is mounted inside the transducer housing in such a way that the face of the transducer array travels along an orbit. The radius was chosen to prevent redundant data acquisition in the nearfield and to assure optimum extension and resolution of the volumetric scan in the farfield. The shape of the coupling interface between the patient body and the 3-D scanhead was developed as a sphere, resulting in an anatomically favorable shape with modest extension.

The chosen accuracy of the stepper motor driving the transducer array enables acquisition of up to three consecutive 2-D images within 1° of sweep (±30° maximum). Immediately after each positioning procedure of the transducer array, the image data is stored digitally (raw data) and then processed as follows. Transformation of each individual pixel from the stored images into a cartesian 3-D coordinate system geometrically reconstructs the ultrasound information of the scanned volume. The coordinates of a single pixel of one 2-D image together with the information of the position of the 2-D image inside the scanned volume determines the corresponding position within the 3-D coordinates. The result of this procedure is a geometrically and spatially correct assignment of the complete ultrasound information (3-D raw data memory).

Up to this point no data reduction or any other kind of postprocessing has been applied to the initially scanned ultrasound information, i.e., no loss of information or image degradation has taken place.

Presentation of the reconstructed three-dimensional data set is performed by projection of the volumetric data or by presentation of user-selectable oblique slices from the 3-D object. The 3-D object can be analyzed through consecutive slices. Distance and orientation of slices are selectable by the user.

In many diagnostic applications the spatial projection of the complete set of 3-D information can provide much higher diagnostic input. The spatial presentation on the monitor of the 3-D workstation is obtained by geometrical perspective projection of all image pixels contained within the 3-D raw data memory.

The following gives a short summary of the algorithm used to present transparent projections for the reconstructed 3-D volume. All projection rays meet in the viewpoint (i.e., the observer's eye), travel through the projection plane (monitor) and intercept the 3-D volume data (see Fig. 4). The number of rays that must be computed results from the number of pixels in the image. The size of this image on the monitor can be determined by the user. The gray-scale value of one pixel at the monitor is calculated from all the 3-D image data intercepted by the corresponding ray. The resulting gray-scale value is a weighted sum of all gray-scale information along a single ray. The corresponding image gives the impression of a transparent 3-D object [2]. To achieve the necessary depth cues, the spatial raw gray-scale values are weighted according to the distance from the observer's eye. To perceive a good spatial impression of the 3-D structure under investigation, the observer's viewpoint is dynamically changed. Through presentation of a precomputed set of coordinated perspective projections in a loop, the impression of a 3-D object rotating in space is achieved. Speed of rotation, distance to object and orientation of object are all user selectable.

Position and extension of the 3-D objects can be recognized and analyzed this way, with improved information content compared to standard 2-D diagnostics.

Throughout the computation process applied to achieve the 3-D presentations, the initially scanned gray-scale values are used as input, i.e., the principle of scaling ultrasound images in gray-scale values common to 2-D imaging is used in the same manner, thus allowing image interpretation according to conventional sonography. Using this approach, the ultrasound-specific presentation characteristic is also maintained throughout the 3-D presentation. Since the complete pixel information belonging to a selected volume of interest is used for calculating the results, no information loss is suffered through processing. This also prevents artifacts and defects in the resulting data, which are nearly unavoidable when manipulating raw data through data reduction, filtering, or manual contouring.

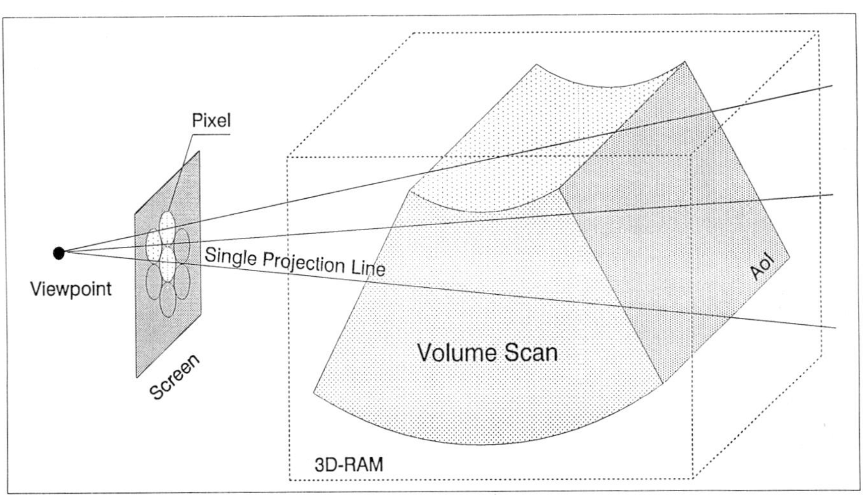

Fig. 4. Principle of transparent, perspective projection

The quality of this kind of presentation depends substantially on the dynamic real-time perception as achieved on the 3-D workstation monitor. The images presented in this chapter, due to their static character, cannot give the same amount of information as a dynamic playback of transparent projections (rotation of 3-D objects). Nevertheless, the static images presented below give an initial impression of the results of initial in vitro and in vivo investigations.

Figure 5 shows four projections from different viewpoints of a branch scanned in a water bath. This branch of a small plant has a very distinct 3-D characteristic and therefore serves well as a test object to study the results of the algorithm used. Outlined with thin white borders is the volume of interest chosen for scanning. During dynamic replay of a rotation sequence this outlining gives additional information concerning orientation and extension of the object under investigation.

Figure 6 presents the results of another in vitro experiment. Shown here are four projections of an excised pork kidney scanned in a water bath.

Figure 7 shows an example of an in vivo volumetric scan performed on a patient awaiting gallstone treatment. Again, four different projections taken from different viewpoints are presented. The upper right projection of Fig. 7, even in this static image, clearly shows the gallbladder containing at least two concrements. Precise localization of stones in kidneys and gallbladders is vital to lithotripsy procedures, and a method similar to the one described here could greatly improve 3-D localization of stones and concrements. Furthermore, exact calculation of stone mass and distribution of concrements at different stages of disintegration could be very valuable when performing lithotripsy procedures.

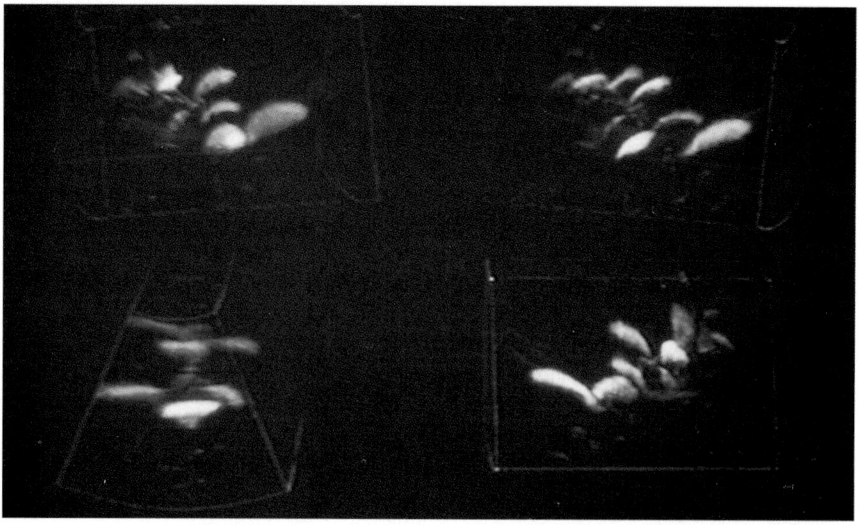

Fig. 5. Four projections of a plant in water bath (in vitro)

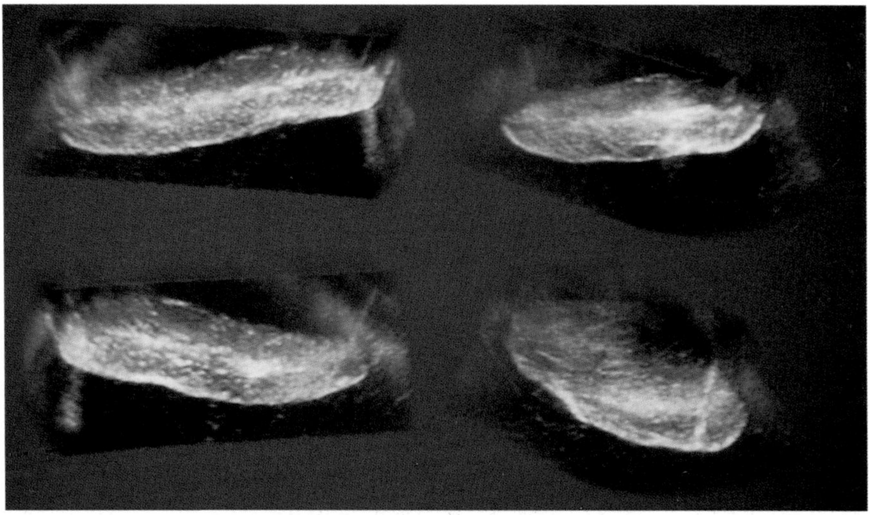

Fig. 6. Four projections of pork kidney (in vitro)

Figure 8 shows the results of a volumetric scan performed on a 15-week-old fetus in vivo. The data presented here were scanned at the Universitätsklinikum Essen, FRG (Dr. Sohn). Again, these static images give a very poor representation of the results compared to the dynamic rotation on the system monitor of the 3-D workstation. However, it is possible to recognize the fetus' head at the bottom of the presented volume, the spine stretching from bottom

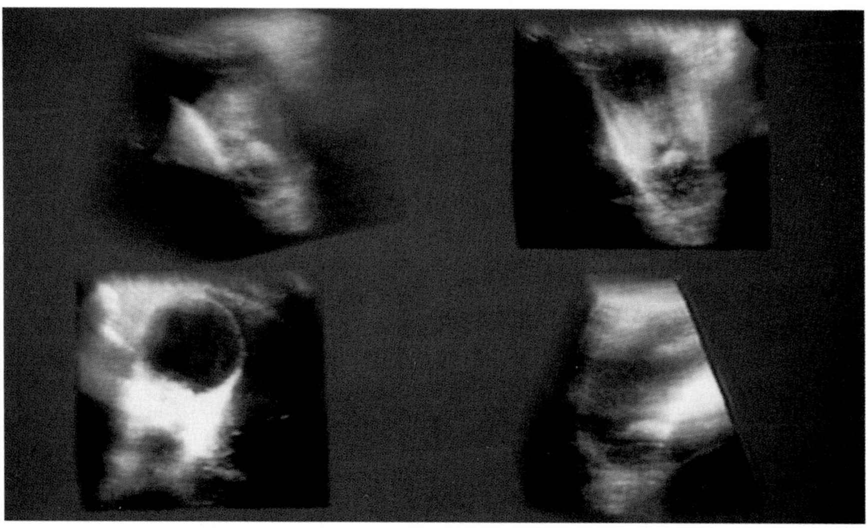

Fig. 7. Four projections of gallbladder with stone (in vivo)

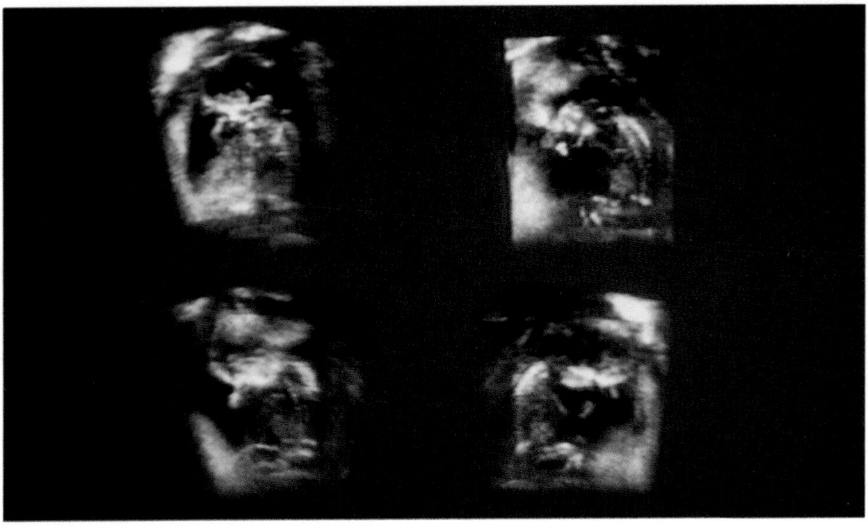

Fig. 8. Four projections of fetus, 15th week (in vivo) (data acquired at Universitätsklinikum Essen; Dr. Sohn)

to top, the hip area, and the knee joints. Our initial clinical results promise a very valuable tool for malformation diagnosis with respect to morphologically visible alterations at very early stages of pregnancy.

Common to all possible applications of this 3-D procedure is the expansion from the strictly 2-D comprehension of structures and shapes in today's 2-D ultrasound imaging to a truely 3-D interpretation. A main interest in many applications consists in the exact quantitative calculation of volumes and the precise localization and shape determination of structures, both practicable only with a geometrically precise 3-D data set. Possible applications can be expected in tumor diagnostics, surgery and radiation planning, volume calculation of organs and arteriosclerotic plaques, fetal malformation diagnosis, and improved biopsy guidance. Further clinical trials will be required to establish the effectiveness and validity of the described procedure as well as to evaluate additional applications.

References

1. Hottier F, Billon AC (1990) 3D echography: status and perspective. In: Höhne KH, Fuchs H, Pizér SM (eds) 3-D imaging in medicine. Springer, Berlin Heidelberg New York, pp 21–41 (NATO ASI Series F, vol 60)
2. La Louche RC, Bickmore D, Mankovich NJ (1989) Three-dimensional reconstruction of ultrasound images. In: The UCLA PACS modules and related projects – a progress report. Available from Medical Imaging Division, Department of Radiological Sciences, University of California, Los Angeles, p 59

Clinical TNM Cancer Staging with Endosonography

T. L. Tio

Introduction

Endoscopic, nonendoscopic, or endoscopic-guided transintestinal sonography, generally known as endosonography (ES), was developed to improve the diagnostic accuracy of transcutaneous ultrasound (US). Remarkable resolution can be obtained through the use of high-frequency real-time US and by direct contact with the target via the intestinal lumen. This imaging modality was introduced for clinical studies in various centers at the beginning of 1980. The ES interpretation of normal gastrointestinal (GI) echo patterns and of biliopancreatic abnormalities has been established, which allows routine use of ES in the daily clinical setting.

The aim of this chapter is to review the clinical TNM staging [1–4] of GI carcinoma by mean of ES [5–12]. The role of ES in planning the strategy of treatment is discussed.

Instruments

We performed all the ES examinations of the upper GI tract with a prototype or commercially available echoendoscope (Olympus EU-M2 or EU-M3) (Fig. 1). Recently, a smaller echoprobe attached to the video or fiberoptic duodenoscope has become available, which is equipped with a bridge for maneuvering the puncture needle or biopsy forceps during the ES procedure. In the case of stenosis which could not be passed with the instruments, we used a small-caliber nonoptic ultrasonic Aloka instrument. In filiform stenosis of esophageal carcinoma, a catheter echoprobe could be introduced through the biopsy channel of a large-caliber gastroscope into the lumen (Fig. 2).

We performed the ES examinations of the lower GI tract with a nonoptic rigid or flexible ultrasonic instrument, a side-viewing duodenoscope, forward-viewing echocolonoscope (Fig. 3).

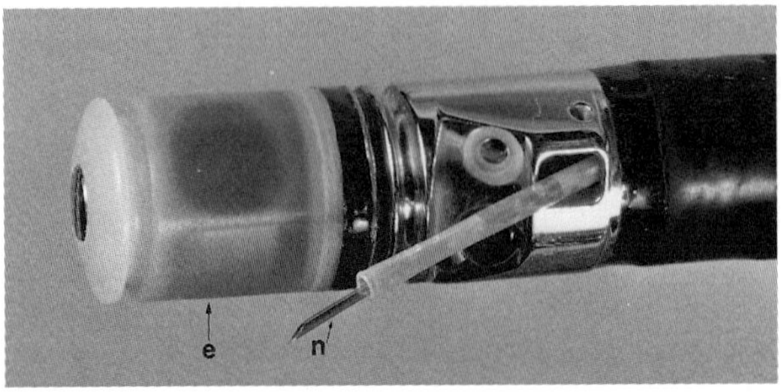

Fig. 1. Echoduodenoscope with a small echoprobe *(e)* attached to the tip of duodenoscope with a modified sclerosing needle *(n)* passing through the biopsy channel

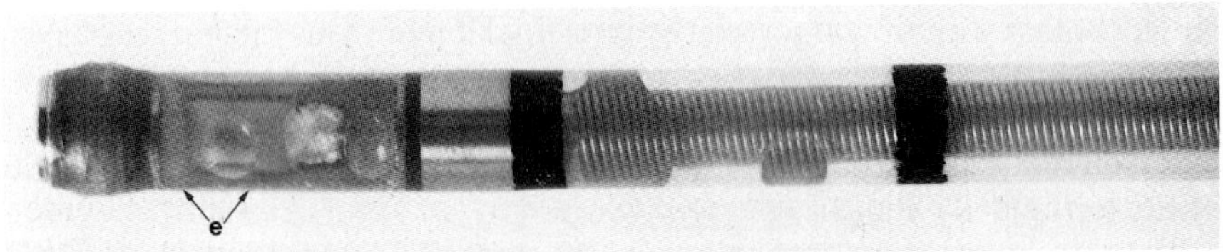

Fig. 2. Olympus catheter echoprobe *(e)* which can be introduced through the biopsy channel of the gastroscope or colonoscope

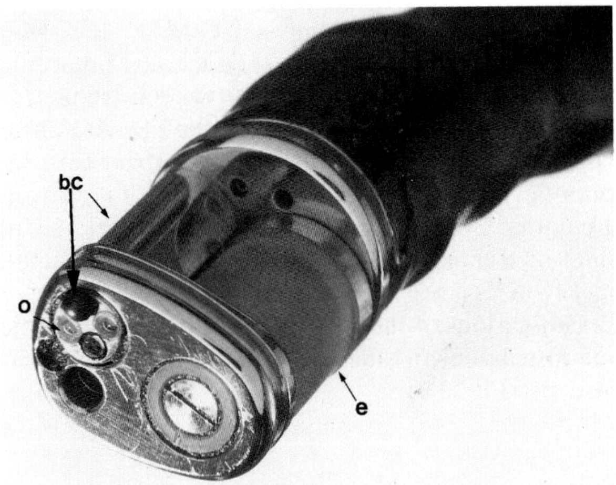

Fig. 3. An echocolonoscope (Olympus XCF-UM2) consisting of a small echoprobe *(e)* attached beyond end-viewing optics *(o)* and parallel to the biopsy channel *(bc)*

Technique of Investigation

Upper GI Tract

Esophagogastric Carcinoma. The investigation technique we used in esophagogastric carcinoma was comparable to routine gastroscopy. Local oropharyngeal anesthesia and intravenous sedation were necessary because of the discomfort to the patient during introduction of the instrument and inflation of the balloon or filling the gastric lumen with water. The echoprobe was positioned adjacent to the target, either endoscopically whenever possible or, on the basis of information gathered during a previous endoscopic examination, with a regular gastroscope. Careful endoscopic measurement of the distance between the teeth and the tumor in the esophagus was mandatory, because the side-viewing optics of the echoendoscope did not permit endoscopic imaging of the lesion in the esophagus. Gastric carcinoma, however, could be localized under endoscopic view. Cross-sectional images comparable to computed tomography (CT) scanning positions were obtained for standarized analysis. Longitudinal and oblique sections were obtained by maneuvering the echoprobe using the desceding aorta or the liver and spleen as landmarks. The latter images were obtained with techniques similar to those used in standard transcutaneous abdominal US. The Japanese nomenclature of regional lymph nodes for the esophagus and stomach could be integrated to permit easier description of various sites of lymph nodes.

Biliopancreatic Carcinoma. The echoprobe was first positioned endoscopically close to the papilla of Vater. Thereafter, the instrument was gradually withdrawn after sonographic imaging of the target lesion (i.e., ampulla, pancreatic head, or distal common bile duct). The extent of the tumor and the regional lymph nodes were carefully assessed using the portal and/or splenic vein or dilated common bile duct as landmarks. The echoprobe was sequentially withdrawn into the duodenal bulb, and antrum and body of the stomach under sonographic control. The right hepatic duct could be imaged from the second part of the duodenum and/or duodenal bulb. The left hepatic duct could be imaged by positioning the echoprobe along the lesser curvature of the stomach, using the left lobe of the liver ans portal vein as landmarks. The image was obtained in the same way as cross-sectional CT scanning positions or transcutaneous abdominal US. Ductulography of the main target should be performed using ERCP in order to accurately assess the site and extend of the tumor. In the case of ampullary carcinoma, lymph nodes at the splenic hilum should be carefully examined because metastatic involvement here is defined as distant metastases.

Lower GI Tract: Colorectal Carcinoma

The technique of investigation we used in the case of colorectal carcinoma was comparable to rectosigmoidoscopy, with patients lying in the left lateral decubitus position after phosphate enema. Rectal digital examination was obligatory to assess the local anatomy and to dilate the anal sphincter muscle prior to insertion of the instrument. The nonoptic instrument was blindly introduced as deeply as possible, and then carefully withdrawn until abnormalities were imaged sonographically. The polypoid or exophytic configuration of tumor could be clearly imaged by filling the rectal lumen with water. In case of proximal colon carcinoma, the lavage that is usually used for routine colonoscopy was necessary. The echoprobe was placed endoscopically, and its position in relation to the target lesion was comparable with that used for examination of the stomach. The echoprobe of the echocolonoscope, however, was attached beyond the forward-viewing optics. Thus, the echoprobe should be inserted approximately 1–2 cm beyond the tumor.

To identify regional lymph nodes and to determine the more proximal noninfiltrated area, the echoprobe should be introduced into the more proximal colon. The instrument can then be gradually withdrawn under sonographic control. The prostate gland, seminal vesicles, bladder, and spine could be used as landmarks. Cross-sectional CT positions should be used for easier interpretation. Various sections of carcinoma, however, should be examined to assess the maximal extent of tumor. Endoscopic biopsy or cytology could be performed through the large biopsy channel. The sector of ES images, however, was only 300° instead of 360° due to the presence of the biopsy channel parallel to the echoprobe.

ES Interpretation

The interpretation of normal and pathological wall and the periintestinal lymph nodes was based on the results obtained through previous studies.

ES classification of the depth of tumor infiltration according to the TNM classification was as follows:

- ES-T1: Hypoechoic tumor located in the mucosa or submucosa
- ES-T2: Hypoechoic tumor located in the mucosa and submucosa extending into the muscularis propria (esophagus) or subserosa (stomach or recto-colon)
- ES-T3: Hypoechoic transmural infiltration penetrating into the adventitia (esophagus), serosa (stomach), or into subserosa and nonperitonealized pericolic or perirectal tissue (rectocolon)
- ES-T4: Deep transmural tumor with penetration into the visceral peritoneum (rectocolon) and/or adjacent structures (esophagus, stomach, or rectocolon)

The tumor categories of ampullary carcinoma were as follows:

- ES-T1: Hypoechoic tumor limited to the ampulla of Vater
- ES-T2: Hypoechoic tumor invading the duodenal wall
- ES-T3: Hypoechoic tumor invading 2 cm or less into the pancreatic parenchyma
- ES-T4: Hypoechoic tumor invading more than 2 cm into the pancreatic parenchyma or other adjacent structures

The tumor categories of pancreatic carcinoma were:

- ES-T1: Hypoechoic tumor limited to the pancreas
  T1a: Tumor 2 cm or less in greatest dimension
  T1b: Tumor more than 2 cm in greatest dimension
- ES-T2: Hypoechoic tumor extending directly to the following: duodenum, bile duct, peripancreatic tissue
- ES-T3: Tumor extending directly to the following: stomach, spleen, colon, adjacent large blood vessels

The tumor categories of extrahepatic bile duct carcinoma were:

- ES-T1: Hypoechoic tumor invading the mucosa or muscle layer
  T1a: Tumor invading only the mucosa
  T1b: tumor invading the muscle layer
- ES-T2: Hypoechoic tumor invading the perimuscular connective tissue
- ES-T3: Hypoechoic tumor invading adjacent structures: liver, pancreas, duodenum, gallbladder, colon, stomach

The criteria for assessing lymph node metastasis with ES were as follows: lymph nodes with hypoechoic pattern and clearly demarcated boundaries were suggestive of malignancy. Direct extension of the primary tumor into adjacent lymph nodes was considered a malignancy. Lymph nodes with hyperechoic (echogenic) pattern and indistinctly demarcated boundaries were considered benign.

ES Findings

Esophageal Carcinoma

In our prospective study involving 74 patients with esophageal carcinoma, ES and CT were carried out to permit preoperative TNM staging. In staging tumor categories, the overall accuracy of ES was 89 % compared with 59 % for CT [5]. The difference between ES and CT was significant ($p < 0.0005$). ES was more accurate than CT in staging early stage carcinomas and nonresectable cancers (Fig. 4). In staging regional lymph node metastases, the overall accuracy of ES was 80 % compared to 51 % for CT. In this series in 26 % of the

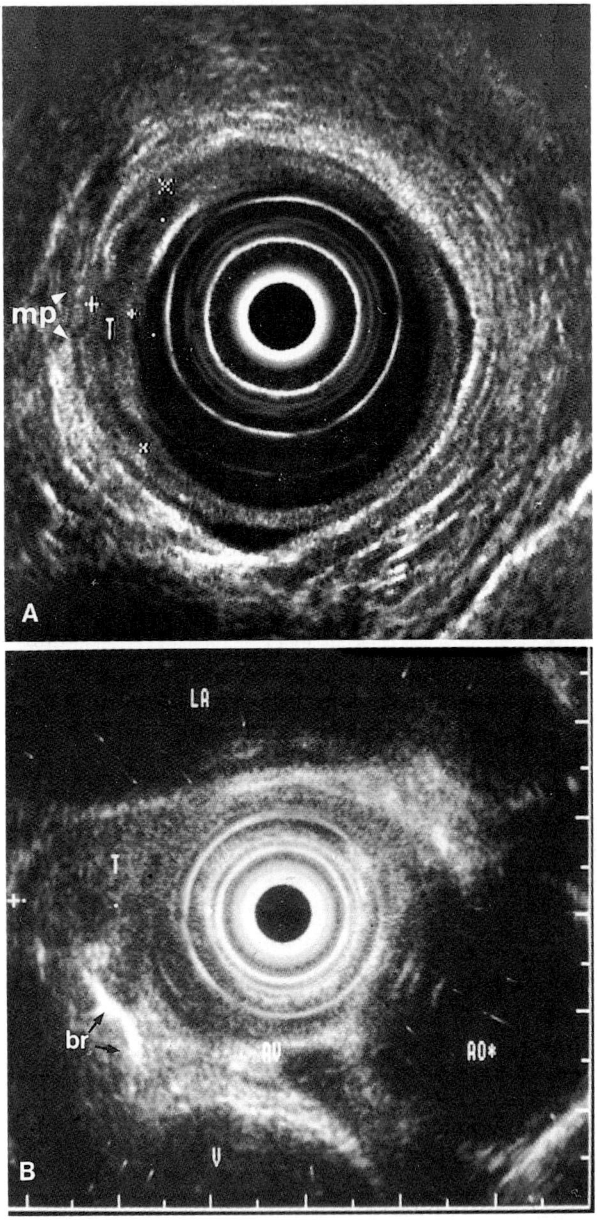

Fig. 4 A, B. Endosonogram reveals **A** a hypoechoic esophageal carcinoma *(t)* located in the mucosa and submucosa without penetration into the muscularis propria *(mp)* compatible with a T1-cancer; and **B** a circular hypoechoic esophageal carcinoma *(t)* with maximal penetration into the right bronchus *(br)*. (*ao*, aorta; *la*, left atrium; *av*, azygos vein; *v*, vertebral)

cases, the stenosis could not be passed with the instrument. In these cases CT was superior to ES in diagnosing celiac lymph node metastases, the overall accuracy of CT being 82 % compared with 68 % for ES. Recently, a catheter echoprobe has become available which can be introduced through the biopsy channel into the stenotic area (Fig. 5). At the Memorial Sloan-Kettering Cancer Center, Lightdale and colleagues carried out a prospective study of preoperative TNM staging of esophageal carcinoma in 50 patients. The results were similar to those of our series. In tumor staging, the accuracy of ES was 92 % compared with 60 % for CT. In N staging, ES accuracy was 88 % compared with 74 % for CT. ES was less accurate in staging distant metastases at 78 % compared with 90 % for CT [6].

Gastric Carcinoma

In our prospective study of 80 patients with gastric carcinoma, the results of ES were similar to those obtained in patients with esophageal carcinoma. The overall accuracy for T staging was 83 % [7, 8]; for N staging, however, the accuracy of ES was only 66 %, due to the difficult anatomical route necessary to identify the entire regional lymph node compared with that taken to identify regional lymph nodes in the esophagus. In the diagnosis of distant metastases, the accuracy of ES was 95 %; the sensitivity, however, was only 33 %, and the specificity 93 %. Peritoneal and liver metastases frequently were not imaged with ES, which explains the low sensitivity rate of ES.

In general, early gastric cancer can be distinguished from an advanced carcinoma on the basis of the depth of tumor penetration. The muscularis propria is clearly visualized as a hypoechoic pattern separating the submucosa from the subserosal layer or perigastric fat tissue. An early gastric cancer is visualized as a T1 carcinoma with or without regional lymph node metastases. Early esophageal carcinoma has been defined as a T1 carcinoma with no evidence of lymph node involvement. Gastric linitis plastics is seen as diffuse submucosal abnormalities with obvious thickening of the infiltrated area associated with thickening of the muscularis propria. If there is intraperitoneal ascites adjacent to the tumor, the serosal layer can be seen as an echogenic layer, representing the second layer after the border echoes produced by the solid – fluid interaction. Thus, a T3 carcinoma can be seen as a hypoechoic tumor infiltrating the outermost echogenic layer adjacent to the ascites (Fig. 6).

Colorectal Carcinoma

In our series of 91 patients with colorectal carcinoma, transintestinal ES was performed using both a nonoptic instrument and an echoendoscope [9]. Both ES and the results of histological examinations of resected specimens were used to stage the carcinomas according to the UICC TNM classification [1].

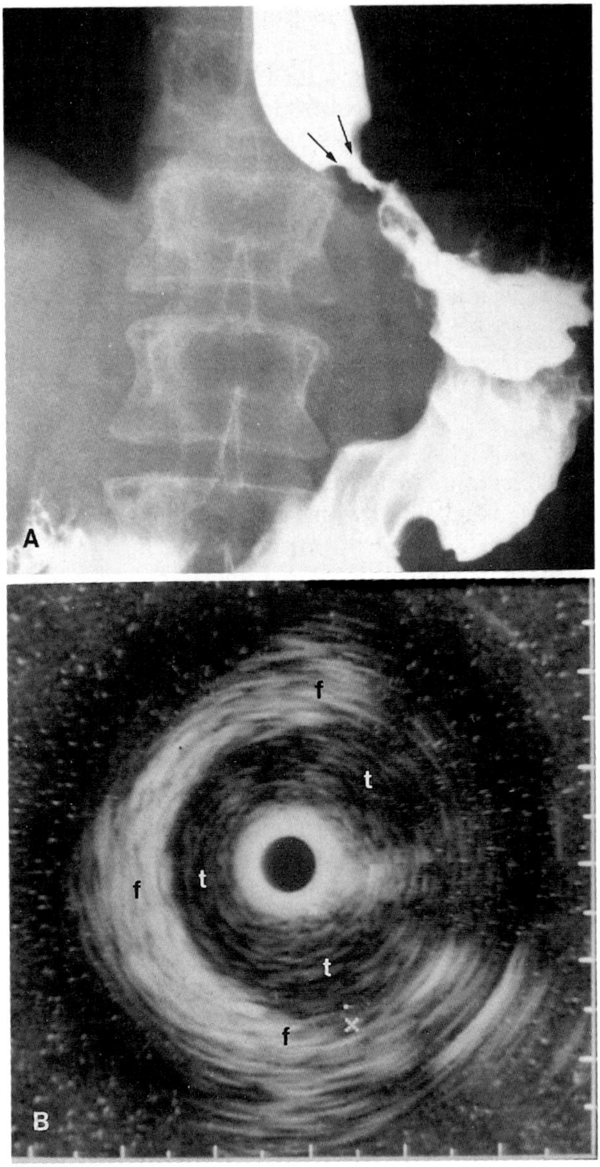

Fig. 5 A. Barium swallow reveals a circular distal esophageal carcinoma with a tight stenosis *(arrows)* which cannot be passed with a gastroscope. **B** A catheter echoprobe introduced via the biopsy channel of gastroscope into the stenotic area reveals a circular hypoechoic tumor *(t)* with penetration into the aventitia *(f)* compatible with a T3 esophageal carcinoma

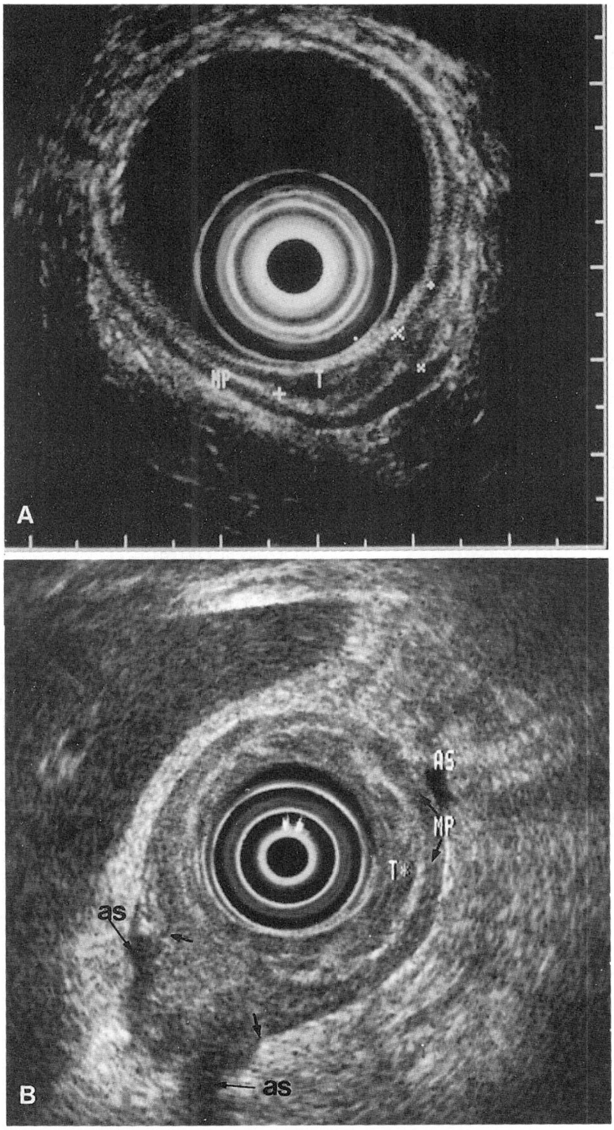

Fig. 6 A, B. Endosonograms showing **A** a hypoechoic cardia tumor *(t)* located in the mucosa *(m)* and submucosa *(sm)* without invading the muscularis propria. The ES diagnosis of early gastric cancer was proven by the histology of resected specimen; and **B** a diffuse submucosal hypoechoic tumor *(t)* with penetration through *(arrows)* the muscularis propria *(mp)* into the serosa. Note the infiltrated serosal layer seen directly adjacent to the ascites *(as)*. The diagnosis of linitis plastica was made due to the diffuse submucosal infiltration with obvious thickening of the infiltrated submucosa and remarkable thickening of the muscularis propria

ES was accurate for all types of tumor staging, except for T2 carcinomas, since because these were accompanied by peritumoral abscess or inflammation overstaging of the tumor resulted on US. Overall, the accuracy of staging rectal and colonic carcinomas was 81 % and 93 % respectively (Fig. 7). Overstaging occurred in 13 % and understaging in 2 % of cases. For regional lymph nodes, the accuracy of ES was 70 %, sensitivity 94 %, and specificity 55 %. Inflammatory lymph nodes were often diagnosed as metastases. The overall accuracy of ES for Dukes classification was only 67 %. The distinction between an early stage carcinoma and advanced cancer could readily be made on the basis of clear imaging of the muscularis propria.

Ampullopancreatic Carcinoma

The major advantage of ES in staging ampullary and pancreatic carcinoma is its ability to distinguish between early stage and advanced cancers in both diseases. Moreover, differentiation between an ampullary tumor and a pancreatic cancer is possible on the basis of the anatomical location of the primary lesion (Fig. 8). In our prospective preoperative TNM staging of 43 patients with pancreatic cancer and 24 patients with ampullary carcinomas, ES was accurate for tumor staging and less accurate for the N classification [10]. The overall accuracy for the T classification in pancreatic and ampullary carcinomas was 92 % and 88 %, respectively. In diagnosing regional lymph node involvement in pancreatic and ampullary carcinomas, the accuracy of ES was 74 % and 54 %, respectively. In predicting lymph node metastases in pancreatic and ampullary carcinomas, the accuracy of ES was 91 % and 80 %, respectively. The prevalence of lymph node metastases in T1 pancreatic cancers and in T1 ampullary carcinomas was 40 % and 0 %, respectively. This figure suggests that early ampullary carcinomas can presumably be treated by local tumor resection (papillectomy) instead of an extensive Whipple procedure [11]. ES may contribute great deal to selecting the appropriate patient for so-called minimally invasive surgery.

Extrahepatic Bile Duct Carcinoma

Extrahepatic bile duct carcinomas have been increasingly reported, probably due to an improvement of diagnositic imaging modalities. The long-term prognosis of this disease has been reported to be unfavorable despite its slow-growing nature and a low incidence of distant metastases. Accurate preoperative staging is essential because the extend of the tumor may be difficult to assess, even at surgery. This is especially true in the case of proximal extrahepatic bile duct carcinomas, the so-called Klatskin tumor, due to its difficult anatomical location and fibrotic appearance on gross macroscopic inspection. Transcutaneous sonography and CT are accurate in diagnosing dilation of bile ducts; however, the extent of and site of the

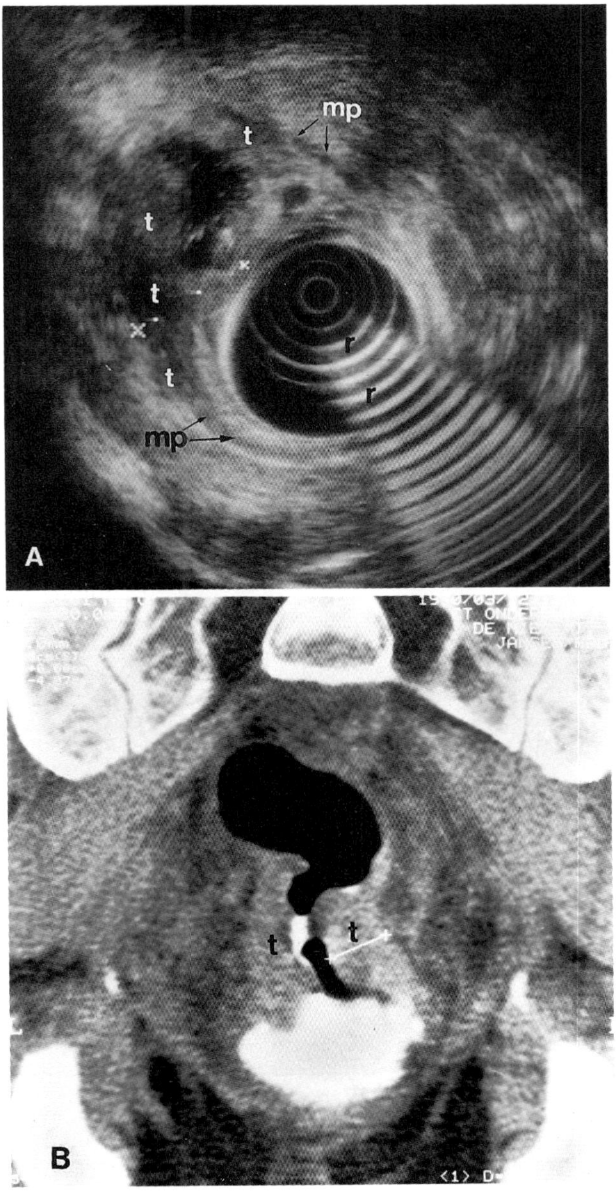

Fig. 7 A. Endosonogram of a transmural hypoechoic rectosigmoid carcinoma with penetration into the perirectal fat tissue compatible with a T3 carcinoma. Note the reverberation phenomen *(r)* due to the biopsy channel adjacent to the echoprobe. **B** Corresponding CT shows a circular wall thickening *(t)* of the rectosigmoid junction. *mp:* muscularis propria

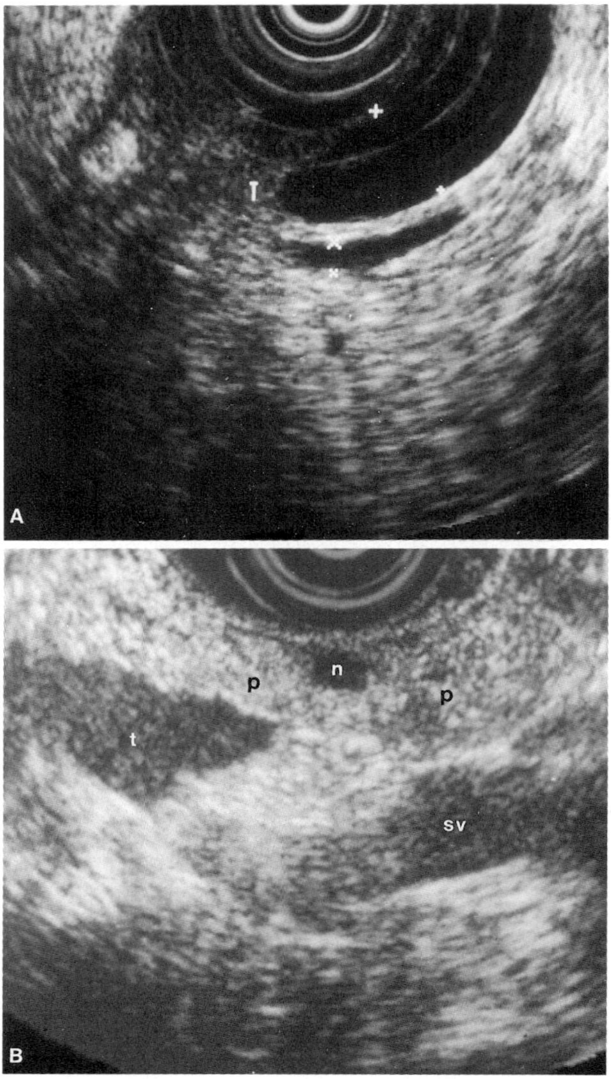

Fig. 8 A, B. Endosonograms revealing **A** an extensive hypoechoic tumor mass *(T)* at the major papilla with penetration into the common bile duct *(t)*, pancreatic duct *(x)* and adjacent pancreas. The extent of the tumor into the pancreas is less than 2 cm in the diameter compatible with a T3 ampullary carcinoma; and **B** a hypoechoic pancreatic tumor *(t)* with penetration into the peripancreatic fibrotic tissue compatible with a T2 pancreatic carcinoma. A small hypoechoic lymph node with sharply demarcated boundaries suggestive of metastasis is seen (*SV,* splenic vein)

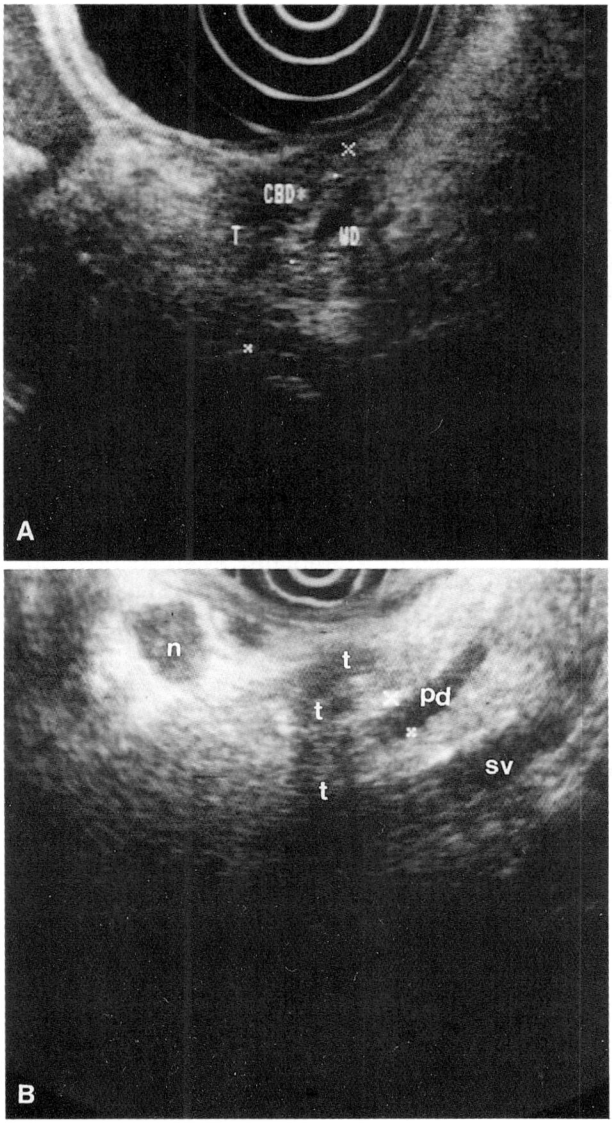

Fig. 9 A, B. Endosonograms showing **A** a transductal hypoechoic common bile duct *(CBP) tumor (t)* with penetration into the periductal pancreatic parenchyma compatible with a T2 bile duct carcinoma (*wd*, Wirsung duct); and **B** a transductal hypoechoic tumor *(t)* with penetration into the adjacent splenic vein *(sv)*. Note the dilated pancreatic duct *(pd)* and a sharply demarcated hypoechoic lymph node *(n)* suggestive of metastasis. The ES findings are compatible with T3N1 carcinoma

primary lesion are more diffucult to image. A prospective study of ES in the preoperative TNM staging of extrahepatic bile duct carcinoma revealed a high accuracy in the tumor staging [12, 13]. The overall accuracy of ES for common bile duct carcinoma and common hepatic duct carcinoma (Klatskin tumor) was 82.8% and 85%, respectively (Fig. 9). ES was helpful in diagnosing regional lymph node metastases, but less accurate in defining nonmetastatic lymph node abnormalities. In the staging of distant metastasis, this technique was limited by the low penetration depth of US. Thus, additional transcutaneous US or CT was necessary for complete staging. In the case of extremely dilated common bile duct, a transpapillary catheter echoprobe could be introduced after papillotomy for endobiliary ES.

Resumé

The main purpose of the TNM classification of carcinoma is to establish accurate clinical staging (cTNM) of the disease. The TNM staging is based on the precise delineation of the local anatomical extent and the spread of the disease to provide a guideline for prognosis and treatment. In staging esophagogastric and colorectal carcinoma, ES is accurate for the assessment of tumor categories due to its ability to image the individual layer of gastrointestinal wall. In the staging of ampullopancreatic and extrahepatic carcinomas, ES is accurate for the tumor staging due to its ability to localize the primary lesion and to image adjacent ductular abnormalities. Thus, ductulography obtained with ERCP or PTC, and parenchymal abnormalities visualized with transcutaneous US can be imaged with ES in one single procedure. Recently, a convex echoendoscope implemented with a color Doppler scanner has become available, which can be used for a combined US-Doppler investigation. Moreover, ES-guided puncture for diagnosis (e.g., submucosal tumor or lymph nodes) or treatment (e.g., pancreas pseudocyst) can be performed because of the continuous imaging of the puncture needle or biopsy forceps during the procedure. In this way, a tissue diagnosis can be obtained during ES procedure which is comparable to endoscopic biopsy. ES can also be performed if a questionable diagnosis has arisen during gastroscopy, colonoscopy, or ERCP. Cancer staging with ES is destined to become a standard procedure in large gastroenterology units.

References

1. Hermanek P, Sobin LH (eds) (1987) TNM classification of malignant tumours. International Union against Cancer, 4th edn. Springer, Berlin Heidelberg New York
2. Sobin LH, Hermanek P, Hutter RP (1988) TNM classification of malignant tumours. Cancer 61: 2310–2314
3. Spiessl B, Beahrs OH, Hermanek P, Hutter RVP, Scheibe O, Sobin LH, Wagner G (eds) (1989) International Union against Cancer TNM Atlas. Springer, Berlin Heidelberg New York

4. Shermann CD, Calman KC, Eckhard S, Elsebai I, et al. (eds) (1987) Manual of clinical oncology. 4th edn. Springer, Berlin Heidelberg New York
5. Tio TL, Cohen P, Coene PP, Udding J, den Hartog Jager FCA, Tytgat GNJ (1989) Preoperative TNM classification of esophageal carcinoma by endosonography and computed tomography. Gastroenterology 96: 1478–1486
6. Lightdale CJ, Bolet JF (1991) Esophageal carcinoma: preoperative staging and evaluation of amastomic recurrence. Gastrointest Endosc 36 [Suppl 2]: S11 – S16
7. Tio TL, Coene PPLO, Schouwink MH, Tytgat GNJ (1989) Esophagogastric carcinoma: preoperative TNM classification with endosonography. Radiology 73: 411–417
8. Tio TL, Schouwink MH, Cikot R, Tytgat GNJ (1989) Preoperative TNM classification of gastric carcinoma by endosonography in comparison with the pathological TNM system: prospective study of 72 cases. Hepatogastroenterology 36: 51–56
9. Tio TL, Coene PPLO, Van Delden OM, Tytgat GNJ (1991) Preoperative TNM classification of colorectal carcinoma by endosonography. Radiology 1979: 165–170
10. Tio TL, Tytgat GNJ, Cikot RJLM, Houthoff HJ (1990) Preoperative TNM classification of pancreatic and ampullary carcinoma by endosonography. Radiology 175: 455–461
11. Tio TL, Mulder CJJ, Eggink WF (1992) Endosonography in staging early carcinoma of the ampulla of Vater. Gastroenterology (in press)
12. Tio TL, Wijers OB, Sars PRA, Tytgat GN (1990) Preoperative TNM classification of proximal extrahepatic bile duct carcinoma by endosonography. Sem Liver Dis 10: 114–120
13. Tio TL, Cheng J, Sars PRA, Tytgat GNJ (1991) Preoperative TNM classification of extrahepatic bile duct carcinoma by endosonography. Gastroenterology 100: 1351–1361

Subject Index

air-filled spheres 2
albumin, human 98, 100
ampullary carcinoma 129, 136
angioplasty, balloon 85
annular array 110
artery 83
– elastic 83
– muscular 83
– plaque 84
ascites, pancreatic 70
azygos vein 61

backscatter 2
– acoustic 1
balloon
– angioplasty 85
– gastroscopy 129
Bauhin's valve 17
bile duct 129, 136
– carcinoma 136
– common 129
biliary tree 39
biodistribution 14
bowel wall 17
bubbles, gaseous micro- 1, 98
Budd-Chiari syndrome 56

C scan 113
carbon dioxide 98
carcinoma
– ampullary 129, 136
– bile duct 136
– colonic 20, 130
– colorectal 130, 133
– – early cancer 87
– esophageal 131
– gastric 36, 129, 133
– – early cancer 133
– hepatocellular 45
– pancreatic 40, 136
– staging 27, 38
– – clinical 41
– – TNM 22, 127
catheter 70, 87
– double-pigtail 70
– flexible 87
cellular dehydration 79
colitis, ulcerative 24
collagen spheres 99
colon 17
– tumor 16, 20
– – carcinoma 20, 130
– – malignancy 41
– – polyps 20
color/colour Doppler 5, 64
color/colour flow mapping 51, 64
colorectal carcinoma 130, 133
compression, extragastric 35
contrast agent 8, 97
– saccharide-based 1
Crohn's disease 24
cyst, pancreatic chronic 70
cystogastrostomy 70

3-D coordinate 122
3-D echography 119
3-D image 110
– pseudo- 113
3-D presentation 119
diagnostic, intraluminal 81
Doppler ultrasound 7
– color/colour imaging 5
– endosonography 67
– – duplex transducer 61
– flowmetry 49, 50
– pulsed 51
– signal enhancement 5
double-pigtail catheter 70
drainage, percutaneous 70
ductulography 129
Dukes classification 136
duodenocystostomy 70
duplex Doppler transducer 61

echo-enhancing 1
echocolonoscope 127
echoduodenoscope 128
echoendoscope 127

elastic artery 83
electronic scanning sonoendoscope 31
endoluminal ultrasound (see also ultrasound) 87, 89, 91, 93
endoscopic ultrasound/endosonography (see also EUS/ES) 27, 28, 34, 61, 67, 127, 133, 140
endourethral transducer 89
esophageal
– carcinoma 131
– malignancy 39
– varices 39, 64
ethanol injection, percutaneous (PEI) 79
EUS/ES (endoscopic ultrasound/endosonography) 27, 61, 127
– Doppler 67
– endobiliary 140
– equipment 28
– indication 34
– transintestinal 133
ex vivo studies 10
extragastric compression 35

fallopian tube 92
five-layer structure 25, 43
flow volume 56

galactose 1
gaseous microbubbles 1, 98
gastric
– lumen 129
– tumor 35
– – carcinoma 36, 129, 133
– – early cancer 133
– – submucosal 35
– varices 38, 61
gastrocystostomy 70
gastrointestinal (GI) tract 16, 127
– carcinome 127
– endoluminal ultrasound 93
gastropathy, hypertensive 61
gastroscope, flexible 88
geometrical resolution 119
gray-scale value 123
gynecological endoluminal ultrasound 91

hepatic veins 55
hepatocellular carcinoma 45
hepatofugal flow 57
human albumin 98
– microspheres 100
hydro-colonic sonography 16
hypertension, portal 51, 55, 62
hypertensive gastropathy 61

IDE (iodipamide ethyl ester) 8, 99
– particles 14
image
– 3-D 110
– intra-arterial 81
– pseudo-3-D 113
inflammatory large-bowel disease 17
instrument, nonoptic 130, 133
interventional vascular methods 81
intestinal lumen 127
intra-arterial imaging 81
intraluminal
– diagnostic 81
– scanning 27
iodipamide ethyl ester (see also IDE) 8, 14, 99

Japanese nomenclature 129

Kupffer's cells 8

laparoscopic ultrasound/ultrasonography 43
layers 25, 34
liver, rabbit 10

mean velocity 56
microbubbles, gaseous 1, 98
microparticles 7
miniaturization 81
muscular artery 83

necroses, acute pancreatic 71
nomenclature, Japanese 129
nonoptic instrument 130, 133

obstetrics, 3-D sonography 110

pancreas 39
pancreatic
– acute necrosis 71
– ascites 70
– carcinoma 40, 136
– chronic cyst 70
– collection of fluid 70
– postacute pseudocyst 71
paraumbilical vein 57
PEI (percutaneous ethanol injection) 79
percutaneous drainage 70
perflourochemicals 99
– perflourocarbon 99
– perflouroctylbromide 99
periesophageal vein 64
phased arrays 82
pigtail catheter, double- 70
plaque, artery 84
polyps, colon 20
portal
– hypertension 51, 55, 62
– pressure 58

- thrombosis 50
- vein 49, 56
projection rays 123
protein denaturation 79
pseudo-3-D image 113
pseudocyst, postacute pancreatic 71
pulmonary transit 1, 2
pulsatility index 53, 55
pulse-echo technique 10

rabbit liver 10
resistance index 53
resolution, geometrical 119
reticuloendothelial system 100
rotating transducer 31

saccharide 1
scanning 27
- intraluminal 27
- transrectal 27
side-viewing optic 129
sonocolonfiberscope 29
sonoendoscopy 27
- electronic scanning 31
sonography, hydro-colonic 16
sonolaparoscope 43
speckle 10
staging carcinoma 27, 38, 136
- clinical 41
- TNM 22, 127
stepper motor 120
stereoscopic inspection 110
stratification, five-layer 25, 43
syndrome, Budd-Chiari 56

three-dimensional (see 3-D)
thrombosis, portal 50
TNM classification 22, 127
transducer 31, 61, 87, 89, 110
- annular array 110
- duplex Doppler 61
- endourethral 89
- miniaturized 87
- rotating 31
transrectal scanning 27
tumor
- colon 16, 20
- gastric submucosal 35
- infiltration 41
- malignant of the stomach 36
- penetration 133
- staging 22, 27, 38, 41, 127, 136

ulcerative colitis 24
ultrasound
- contrast agents 1, 8, 97
- endoluminal 87
- - endourethral 89
- - gastrointestinal use 93
- - gynecological use 91
- laparoscopic 43

varices
- esophageal 39, 64
- gastric 38, 61
vascular methods, interventional 81
vein
- azygos 61
- hepatic 55
- paraumbilical 57
- periesophageal 64
- portal 49, 56
velocity, blood flow 56
- mean 56
- profile 56
videoendoscope 29
volumetric scan 122

wall stratification, five-layer 25, 43

Printing: Saladruck, Berlin
Binding: Buchbinderei Lüderitz & Bauer, Berlin